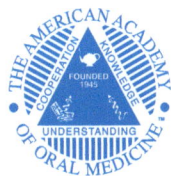

CLINICIAN'S GUIDE
Salivary Gland and Chemosensory Disorders
SECOND EDITION

EDITORS

Michael T. Brennan, DDS, MHS
Director, Sjögren's Syndrome and Salivary Disorders Center
Professor and Chair
Department of Oral Medicine
Carolinas Medical Center
Charlotte, North Carolina

Philip C. Fox, DDS, PC
PC Fox Consulting
Spello, Italy

CONTRIBUTING AUTHORS

Ibtisam Al-Hashimi, BDS, MS, PhD
Joseph A. D'Ambrosio, DDS, MS
Michael T. Brennan, DDS, MHS
Joel B. Epstein, DMD, MSD, FRCD(C)
Beatrice Gandara, DDS, MSD
Miriam Grushka, MSC, DDS, PhD
James Guggenheimer, DDS
Diana V. Messadi, DDS, MMSc, DMSc
Paul A. Moore, DMD, PhD, MPH
Athena Papas, DMD, PhD
Nelson Rhodus, DMD, MPH
Vidya Sankar, DMD, MHS
Mabi Singh, DMD, MS
Medha Singh, BDS, MS
Andrew Spielman, DMD, PhD
Temitope Omolehinwa, BDS
Michael Turner, DDS, MD
Frederick B. Vivino, MD, FACR
Ava Wu, DDS
Fariba S. Younai, DDS

COPY EDITOR

Kathleen A. Sullivan, MA

Most contributing authors are members of the American Academy of Oral Medicine, while others are experts in the fields of dry mouth or chemosensory disorders. This monograph represents a consensus of the contributing authors and not necessarily the private views of any of the individuals.

CONTENTS

American Academy of Oral Medicine
2150 N. 107th St., Suite 205
Seattle, Washington 98133
TEL: (206) 209-5279
EMAIL: info@aaom.com   WEBSITE: www.aaom.com
©2019 American Academy of Oral Medicine

ISBN
print: 978-1-936176-57-1
PDF: 978-1-936176-58-8

Printed in the United States

Notice: The authors and publisher have made every effort to ensure that the patient care recommended herein, including choice of drugs and drug dosages, is in accord with the accepted standard and practice at the time of publication. However, since research and regulation constantly change clinical standards, the reader is urged to check the product information sheet included in the package of each drug, which includes recommended doses, warnings, and contraindications. This is particularly important with new or infrequently used drugs. Any treatment regimen, particularly one involving medication, involves inherent risk that must be weighed on a case-by-case basis against the benefits anticipated. The reader is cautioned that the purpose of this book is to inform and enlighten; the information contained herein is not intended as, and should not be employed as, a substitute for individual diagnosis and treatment.

ABOUT THE AMERICAN ACADEMY OF ORAL MEDICINE (AAOM): The AAOM is a 501c6; nonprofit organization founded in 1945 as the American Academy of Dental Medicine and took its current name in 1966. The members of the American Academy of Oral Medicine include an internationally recognized group of health care professionals and experts concerned with the oral health care of patients who have complex medical conditions, oral mucosal disorders, and / or chronic orofacial pain. Oral Medicine is the field of dentistry concerned with the oral health care of medically complex patients and with the diagnosis and non-surgical management of medically-related disorders or conditions affecting the oral and maxillofacial region.

AMERICAN ACADEMY OF ORAL MEDICINE

MISSION:

1. To promote the study and dissemination of knowledge of the medical aspects of dentistry while serving the best interests of the public.

2. To promote the highest standards of care in the diagnosis and treatment of oral conditions that are not responsive to conventional dental or oral maxillofacial surgical procedures.

3. To provide an avenue of referral for dental practitioners who have patients with severe, life- threatening medical disorders or complex diagnostic problems involving the oral and maxillofacial region that require ongoing nonsurgical management.

4. To improve the quality of life of patients with medically related oral disease.

5. To foster increased understanding and cooperation between medical and dental professions.

6. To obtain American Dental Association recognition of oral medicine as a specialty.

The Academy achieves these goals by holding national meetings annually; by presenting lectures, workshops, and seminars; by sponsorship of the American Board of Oral Medicine; by the editorship of the Oral Medicine Section of *Oral Surgery, Oral Medicine, Oral Pathology, Oral Radiology*, and *Endodontics*; and by publishing monographs and position papers on timely subjects relating to oral medicine.

The presented information is based on current knowledge and accepted standards of practice. Following the guidelines set forth in this monograph may not ensure successful management of every patient. This monograph represents a con-sensus of the editors and authors and not necessarily the private views of any individual.

All brand name medications may have patents, service marks, trademarks, or registered trademarks and are the property of their respective companies.

This Clinician's Guide is another AAOM educational service.
Other Clinician's Guides available from the Academy include:

Treatment of Common Oral Conditions
Tobacco Cessation
Oral Health in Geriatric Patients
Chronic Orofacial Pain
Medically Complex Dental Patients

Preface

Thank you for the purchase of the AAOM monograph: Clinician's Guide to Salivary Gland and Chemosensory Disorders. This publication is the culmination of a great deal of work from a wide array of authors, including a number of world leaders and widely recognized educators in their respective areas of contribution. The real challenge for us as editors has been to condense the tremendous volume of their expertise into a manageable and succinct publication without sacrificing any of the valuable information they provided. We can only hope we have succeeded in a way that does justice to the considerable time and effort they have so generously volunteered to this project.

Xerostomia is defined as the sensation of oral dryness. It is a common symptom but does not constitute a diagnostic entity; this subjective patient report may or may not be associated with a significant alteration in salivary function. Xerostomia may be experienced as a result of altered oral sensory function, changes in composition or viscosity of saliva, and/or reductions in stimulated or unstimulated salivary output. When xerostomia is a result of salivary alterations, a general diagnosis of salivary gland dysfunction (or hypofunction) may be made. With evaluation, if a more specific etiology is identified, the diagnosis should reflect that information (such as a diagnosis of radiation-induced salivary gland dysfunction).

All recommended treatments were current at the time of the publication of this guide. However, new medications are constantly made available to the clinician and therapeutic strategies evolve with new knowledge. The prudent clinician is well advised to consider this when using this guide.

Some of the recommended treatments have been more thoroughly investigated than others, but all have been reported to be of clinical value. For many conditions described in this monograph, there is currently no cure, but there are treatment modalities that can relieve discomfort, shorten the clinical duration and frequency, and minimize sequelae.

Once again, thank you for your purchase of this AAOM Clinician's Guide to Salivary Gland and Chemosensory Disorders. We hope that it is a useful addition to your reference library and welcome suggestions for alterations and additions that may be incorporated into future editions.

Michael Brennan and Philip Fox, Editors

Standard Abbreviations

I	One	Prn	as needed (pro re nata)
ii	Two	Q	Every
iii	Three	q2h	every 2 hours
a	Before	q4h	every 4 hours
ac	before meals (ante cibum)	q6h	every 6 hours
ad lib	as desired (ad libitum)	q8h	every 8 hours
asap	as soon as possible	q12h	every 12 hours
AAOM	American Academy of Oral Medicine	Qam	every morning
bid	twice a day (bis in die)	Qd	every day (quaque die)
btl	Bottle	Qhs	every bedtime
c	With	Qid	four times a day (quarter in die)
cap	Capsule	Qod	every other day
CBC	complete blood count	Qpm	every evening
CDC	U.S. Center for Disease Control and Prevention	qsad	add a sufficient quantity to equal
crm	Cream	qwk	every week
disp	dispense on a prescription label	RAS	recurrent aphthous stomatitis
elix	Elixir	RAU	recurrent aphthous ulcer
FDA	U.S. Food and Drug Administration	RBC	red blood cell count
g	Gram	RHL	recurrent herpes labialis
gtt	Drop	RIH	recurrent intraoral herpes
h	Hour	Rx	Prescription
hs	at bedtime	s	Without
HSV	herpes simplex virus	Sig	patient dosing instructions on prescription label
IU	international units	Sol	Solution
IV	Intravenous	SPF	sun protection factor
L	Liter	stat	Immediately
liq	Liquid	Syr	Syrup
loz	Lozenge	Tab	Tablet
mg	Milligram	tbsp	Tablespoon
min	Minute	Tid	three times a day (ter in die)
mL	Milliliter	Top	Topical
NaF	sodium fluoride	Tsp	Teaspoon

Standard Abbreviations (continued)

Oint	Ointment	U	Unit
OTC	over-the-counter	ut dict	as directed (ut dictum)
Oz	Ounce	UV	Ultraviolet
P	After	Visc	Viscous
Pc	after meals	VZV	varicella-zoster virus
PABA	para-aminobenzoic acid	WBC	white blood cell count
PHN	postherpetic neuralgia	Wk	Week
PLT	platelet count	Yr	Year
Po	by mouth (per os)	Zn	Zinc

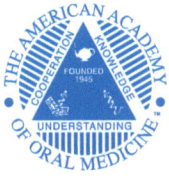

1 Xerostomia: Causes, Symptoms, and Signs

Causes (Etiology)

Xerostomia is the subjective perception of oral dryness. Although it is usually associated with dysfunction of the salivary glands, a complaint of dry mouth is not always a result of reduced production of saliva. Furthermore, the oral tissues may be moist even though some patients complain of dryness. Conversely, patients who have developed clinical manifestations of reduced saliva may not be aware of or complain of xerostomia.

Non-salivary causes of xerostomia include oral sensory alterations, cognitive deficiencies and psychological factors. Xerostomia also may be the consequence of qualitative changes in saliva.

In terms of common etiologic factors, pharmaceuticals are the most prominent cause of xerostomia (Table 1). Table 2 lists other factors often associated with xerostomia including Sjögren's syndrome treatment for thyroid cancer with radioactive iodine (^{131}I), and radiation therapy for head and neck malignancies.

Drug-induced Xerostomia

The following should be noted about medication-induced xerostomia:

- Many commonly prescribed medications have been reported to cause xerostomia (Table 1).
- Different pharmacologic categories of drugs can have xerostomic (xerogenic) effects (Table 1).

The use of medications increases with age. Almost 90% of persons aged 65 and older take at least one prescription medication and 39% take five (5) or more prescription drugs. Consequently, the likelihood of medication-induced xerostomia will continue to increase in conjunction with increasing life expectancy. The reduced metabolism and bodily function may cause more drug availability and cause more salivary hypofunction.

TABLE 1: DRUGS ASSOCIATED WITH XEROSTOMIA		
Pharmacologic Category	*Mode of Action*	*Example*
Antianxiety	Benzodiazepine	Alprazolam
Anticonvulsant	CNS neurotransmitter inhibitor	Gabapentin
Antidepressants	Dopamine/norepinephrine- reuptake inhibitor	Bupropion
	MAO inhibitor	Tranylcypromine
	Selective norepinephrine reuptake inhibitor	Venlafaxine
	SSRI	Fluoxetine
	SSRI/antagonist	Trazadone
	Tricyclic	Amitriptyline
Antidiarrheal	Anticholinergic	Atropine

Table 1 continues on next page ➡

TABLE 1: DRUGS ASSOCIATED WITH XEROSTOMIA *(continued)*		
Pharmacologic Category	**Mode of Action**	**Example**
Antiemetic	Histamine H1 antagonist	Meclizine
Antihypertensives	Alpha2-adrenergic agonist	Clonidine
	Alpha1 blocker	Doxazosin
Antimanic, antipsychotic	Phenothiazine antipsychotic	Chlorpromazine
Antimigraine	Ergot alkaloid	Ergotamine
	Serotonin 5-HT$_{1B,1D}$ receptor agonist	Sumatriptan
Antineoplastic agents	Immunomodulators	Interferons
	Retinoic acid derivative	Tretinoin
	Iodine radioiosotope	^{131}I
Anti-Parkinson's	Anticholinergic	Benztropine
	Dopamine agonist	Amantadine
	MAO type B inhibitor	Rasagline
Antispasmotics	Anticholinergic	Mepenzolate
	Smooth muscle relaxant	Oxybutynin
Antitussive	Antihistamine	Chlorpheniramine
Antivirals (Anti-Hepatitis C virus)	Nucleoside antiviral	Ribavirin
	Interferon alpha-2b	Interferon
Appetite stimulant/antiemetic	Synthetic cannabinoid	Dronabinol
Benign prostatic hyperplasia	Alpha$_1$ adrenergic blocker	Tamsulosin
Bronchodilator	Sympathomimetic β$_2$-agonist	Albuterol
CNS stimulant	Sympathomimetic	Methamphetamine
Decongestant	Sympathomimetic α$_1$ agonist	Phenylephrine
Expectorant	Sympathomimetic	Ephedrine
Gastric acid inhibitor	Proton pump inhibitors	Esomeprazole
Histamine H1 antagonist	Antihistamine	Fexofenadine
Hypnotic	Selective GABA inhibitor	Zolpidem
Immunosuppressant	Calcineurin inhibitor	Cyclosporine
Muscle relaxant	Skeletal muscle relaxant	Cyclobenzaprine
Opioid analgesic	Opioid	Codeine
Overdose antidote	Opioid antagonist	Naltrexone
Smoking cessation	Nicotine	Nicotine-containing products
	Nicotine agonist	Varenicycline
	Antidepressant	Bupropion

Key points to consider when medication-induced xerostomia is encountered:

- Most drugs with xerostomic side-effects are not known to cause permanent damage to the salivary glands.
- Drug-induced xerostomia will resolve when the medication is discontinued. Nevertheless, a majority of xerogenic medications are used to treat chronic conditions. This makes it more likely that the salivary hypofunction will persist.
- Saliva substitutes can relieve the unpleasant symptoms of xerostomia, but the adverse effects of salivary hypofunction on the dentition and oral mucosa may require definitive therapeutic interventions.

TABLE 2: SYSTEMIC CONDITIONS WITH ASSOCIATED XEROSTOMIA
Sjögren's syndrome (see Chapter 4)
Radiation-induced xerostomia
Related to radiation treatment for head and neck malignancies
Dehydration associated with fever, low fluid intake, diarrhea or polyuria, high salt intake
Depression, anxiety or stress
Hepatitis C
HIV
Graft vs. host disease
Sarcoidosis
Chronic Fatigue Syndrome; Fibromyalgia
Nutritional Disorders (e.g., anorexia nervosa)
Alcoholism
Diabetes

Xerostomia Associated with Systemic Disease

Most conditions are associated with a reduction in salivary flow, which affects more than a single salivary gland (Table 2).

SYMPTOMS

- Patients may complain of dryness of the mouth (especially at night when salivary flow is normally at its lowest) or soreness of the mouth.
- Patients also may complain of a chronic burning sensation and intolerance to spicy foods.
- Halitosis may also be reported/experienced by patients with an oral dryness complaint.
- Hyposalivation can lead to serious negative effects on an individual's quality of life; affecting dietary habits, nutritional status, speech, taste, andtolerance to dental prostheses

SIGNS

- Signs of salivary gland dysfunction include mucosal erythema with a "parched" appearance, atrophy of the tongue papillae with fissuring, dry or cracked lips, thick frothy saliva, no salivary pooling on the floor of the mouth, accumulation of plaque, gingivitis, oral infections (particularly candidiasis), mucous plug, sialolithiasis, recurrent parotitis or chronic salivary gland enlargement, dental caries, tooth surface loss (e.g., erosion, attrition, abrasion) and tooth loss.
- It may be difficult to chew and swallow dry foods such as biscuits and crackers

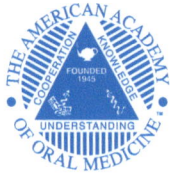

2 Xerostomia: Diagnosis

Diagnosis of salivary gland dysfunction is based on history, clinical examination and specific diagnostic tests.

History

- Past medical history should focus on those conditions and medications known to cause xerostomia.
- Certain subjective complaints (Table 3) have been shown to be associated with quantitative reductions in salivary function.

Examination Findings Include:

- Dry and cracked lips
- The oral mucosa may appear dry and shiny/glassy appearance
- Food debris may stick to teeth or soft tissue and the normal pooling of saliva in the floor of mouth is absent
- Demineralization of teeth and carious lesions may be seen on the cervical margins or neck of the teeth (class V), incisal margins and cusp tips (class VI)
- The tongue may become fissured or have loss of papillation.
- Clinical manifestations of candidiasis, most commonly characterized by angular cheilitis, mucosal erythema and white adherent plaques. Erythematous candidiasis may be more common than more readily recognized pseudomembranous candidiasis (thrush) in patients with salivary hypofunction
- Enlarged salivary glands or masses in the glands
- Palpation of the parotid gland and milking of the gland and duct may reveal little or no saliva output, a thicker/cloudy saliva, or purulent discharge associated with recurrent infections of the salivary glands
- Patients may also report dryness of the eyes, which is suggestive of Sjögren's syndrome

Determination of Salivary Function

- Salivary flow rates can be determined by collection of whole saliva or individual gland output. Both resting and stimulated secretions may be obtained. Whole saliva collection is a simple procedure, which can be accomplished in the dental office. Individual gland secretions require specialized equipment and expertise.
- Unstimulated whole saliva flow rates are determined by allowing passive collection of saliva in the mouth with expectoration of the contents every minute for 5 to 15 minutes. The subject must have been NPO and without any oral stimulation for at least 2 hours prior

TABLE 3: QUESTIONNAIRE FOR SUBJECTIVE EVALUATION OF XEROSTOMIA	
Question	**Response**
Do you have difficulties swallowing any foods?	Yes / No
Does your mouth feel dry while eating a meal?	Yes / No
Do you sip liquids to aid in swallowing dry foods?	Yes / No
Does the amount of saliva in your mouth seems to be too little, too much, or you don't notice it?	Too little/don't notice or/too much
The first response to each of these questions is significantly associated with reduced salivary output in xerostomia patients	

to the examination. For stimulated whole salivary flow, the patient chews on a small piece of paraffin wax or gum base for 5 to 15 minutes and all the saliva is collected into a pre-weighed graduated tube or vial. Saliva volume can be estimated by weight, as 1 mL of saliva weighs approximately 1 g. Therefore, a collection of 1 g in 1 min can be assumed to be equivalent to a salivary flow rate of 1 mL/min.

- Values of <0.1mL/min for unstimulated and <0.7mL/min for stimultated whole salivary flow are considered abnormal and consistent with salivary hypofunction. It is generally accepted that when glandular fluid production is decreased by about 50%, a person will have symptoms of dry mouth.

Salivary Biopsy

Biopsy of labial minor salivary glands or parotid glands is useful in diagnosis of immune-mediated gland dysfunction. A salivary gland biopsy may also indicate other conditions such as granulomatous diseases, amyloidoisis and graft versus host disease. Fine needle aspiration cytology or open biopsy of salivary gland lesions may be needed for evaluation of cysts, lumps and lesions suspected of malignancy.

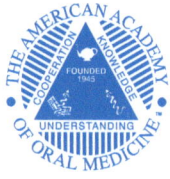

3 Xerostomia: Management

Rationale for Treatment

The mouth is a complex dynamic organ essential for communication, nourishment, and social life; salivary function is important to facilitate these functions. Reduction in salivary output and change in saliva quality is associated with increased incidence of oral diseases, compromised oral function, and may have overwhelming impact on the patient's quality of life. Restoring salivary flow is essential for optimal oral health and minimizing the risk for oral diseases.

CONSIDERATIONS FOR TREATING DRUG-INDUCED HYPOSALIVATION

Determine the xerostomia prevalence rate of patient's medications

- Patients taking multiple xerogenic agents are more likely to report dry mouth symptoms
- Symptoms are most common among older patients
- Assess severity of hyposalivation by measuring unstimulated and stimulated salivary flow rates
- Consult patient's physician regarding alternative medications

CONSIDERATIONS FOR TREATING RADIATION-INDUCED HYPOSALIVATION

Intensity modulated radiotherapy (IMRT) can decrease radiation exposure to individual major salivary glands.

- Use of radioprotective agents such as amifostine may provide cytoprotection to the gland tissue

CONSIDERATIONS FOR TREATING AUTOIMMUNE MEDIATED HYPOSALIVATION

- Understand medical diagnosis
- Assess severity of hyposalivation by measuring unstimulated and stimulated salivary flow rates

Treatments

For the patient with drug-induced xerostomia, substitution of causative medications with similar types of medication with fewer xerostomic side effects should be considered, whenever applicable. For example, serotonin specific re-uptake inhibitors (SSRIs) have been reported to cause less dry mouth than tricyclic antidepressants. Use of anticholinergic drugs only during the daytime may minimize the symptoms at night. Also, division of dosage may reduce the side effects of a single large dose.

The management of general xerostomia symptoms should begin with identification and management of the underlying cause(s) when possible. Current treatment approaches for xerostomia are directed towards providing symptomatic relief and prevention of associated complications. Treatment of xerostomia falls into three basic categories: mechanical (chewing gum), topical (artificial lubricants and mouth rinses) and systemic (Tables 4 & 5). The prevention of negative effects on oral health due to hyposalivation is vital. Establishing the presence of residual salivary gland function by salivary flow rates helps guide treatment management strategies for dry mouth. A patient with a low unstimulated and a similarly low stimulated flow represents poor residual salivary gland function and treatments results may vary.

Salivary stimulation is the preferred treatment in patients with residual salivary gland function. Saliva secretion may be increased by non-specific mechanical and gustatory stimulants. The combination of stimulation by chewing and taste, such as provided by gums and lozenges, can be effective in relieving symptoms. Use of citric acid can stimulate salivation, but its use is limited by mucosal irritation in edentate patients and the risk of demineralization in patients with teeth. Sugar free, xylitol containing chewing gums and candies are useful in patients with residual salivary function. Not all patients will be able to tolerate frequent gum chewing as this may exacerbate temporomandibular disorder (TMD) symptoms.

TABLE 4: XEROSTOMIA MANAGEMENT – NON-SYSTEMIC STRATEGIES

Minimize aggravating factors
    Medication substitution
    Avoid alcohol and other irritants
    Avoid smoking and low-humidity conditions
    Correct mouth breathing
    Treat oral candidiasis
    Avoid tartar control toothpastes
Simple corrective measures
    Liberal use of fluids
    Dietary modification
    Room air humidifier
Gustatory stimulation–Sugar free candies (mild/fruit flavor)
Mechanical stimulation–Sugar free chewing gum (mild/fruit flavor)
Salivary substitutes*–May be helpful for patients who cannot tolerate pharmacologic agents in patients with residual gland function: NOTE–these are examples only with other products available
    COLGATE® HYDRIS™ DRY Mouthwash (Colgate-Palmolive Company)
    Entertainer's Secret® (KLI Corp) spray
    Lubricity® Spray (You First Services)
    MighTeaFlow ® Dry Mouth Rinse, Spray (Camellix)
    Moi-Stir (Kingswood Laboratories)
    Moisyn Advanced Formula for Dry Mouth Relief Rinse & Spray (Prisyna)
    Mouth-Kote®** (Parnell Pharmaceuticals)
    Oral Balance® (Laclede Professional Products)
    OraCoat XyliMelts Dry Mouth Discs (OraHeath)
    SALIVEA™ Dry Mouth Care Products (Laclede, Inc.)
    SalivaSure™ (Scandinavian Natural Health & Beauty) tablets
  * Salivary substitutes are OTC and they can be used as needed; there is no limit for total daily intake
  ** Contains citric acid and could potentially cause softening of the teeth

TABLE 5: XEROSTOMIA MANAGEMENT – SYSTEMIC TREATMENTS

Pharmacologic salivary stimulants (Require Prescription)
    Salagen (Pilocarpine HCl), MGI Pharma, Inc.
    Evoxac (Cevimeline HCl), Daiichi Pharmaceutical Co. Ltd.
Examples of prescriptions
    Rx: Pilocarpine HCl (Salagen)* Tablets 5 mg
    Disp: 90 Tablets
    Sig: Take 1 tablet qid with food.
    Rx: Cevimeline (Evoxac)* Capsules 30 mg
    Disp: 90 Tablets
    Sig: Take 1 tablet tid
* *May require several months to determine effectiveness*
* *Start at 1x/day and titrate the dosing frequency up as tolerated*
* *Avoid in patients with narrow angle glaucoma and uncontrolled asthma*
* *Caution in hypertensive patients who are using ß-blocker*

If saliva secretion cannot be stimulated, symptomatic treatment involves mucosal comfort agents such as saliva substitutes, rinses or sprays. Patients should be encouraged to take frequent sips of fluids throughout the day to hydrate the mucosa. Use of liquid during meals can help in swallowing and improving taste perception. Commercially available saliva substitutes containing thickening agents such as carboxymethyl cellulose and mucin are the most common. Recently, saliva substitutes based upon polymer chemistry have been developed. Cetylpyridinium chloride (CPC) and glycerine based oral rinses may improve the moisturizing effect. While there is clearly a role for the use of saliva replacements, particularly in individuals who have no residual salivary gland function, it must be recognized that this is not a highly effective symptomatic therapy. Also, the pH of these products must be considered to preserve the integrity of tooth structures. Use of bedside humidifiers, particularly at night, may lessen discomfort due to oral dryness.

Systemic Treatments for Xerostomia

Systemic treatments have the benefit of increasing production of a patient's own saliva and its beneficial components. Currently, approved systemic treatments are Salagen (pilocarpine), a nonselective muscarinic agent, and Evoxac (cevimeline). Potential side effects include sweating, chills, nausea, dizziness, rhinitis and asthenia. Cevimeline is said to have an affinity towards M3 receptors of the salivary glands and lower affinity for the M2 receptors of the heart, theoretically leading to less side effects. These drugs may be prescribed in consultation with the patient's physician due to their potential side effects. The dosages of each can be adjusted (titrated) to that which increases saliva while minimizing side effects. Cevimeline has longer duration of effect (approximately 5 hours) compared with pilocarpine (3 hours). Importantly, these medications work best in patients who have some residual salivary gland function. Systemic pilocarpine has the added benefit of increasing eye comfort in dry eye patients with Sjögren's syndrome (SS). Interestingly, a topical preparation of pilocarpine, in the form of a mouth rinse, has been shown to be effective in increasing salivary flow without systemic adverse effects. These agents may be most useful in patients who maintain the ability to produce some amount of saliva.

In conditions where saliva production is limited due to an underlying inflammatory condition (i.e., SS or HCV), the following agents may be beneficial. Omega-3s from dietary consumption are elongated by enzymes to produce anti-inflammatory prostaglandin E3 (PGE3) and anti-inflammatory leukotrine B5 (LTB5). Even more importantly, eicosapentaenoic acid (EPA), a long-chain omega-3 provided directly by fish oils, blocks the gene expression of the pro-inflammatory cytokines tumor necrosis factor alpha (TNF-α), interleukin-1α (IL-1α), interleukin-1b (IL-1b), proteoglycan degrading enzymes (aggrecanases) and cyclooxygenase (COX-2). The consumption of omega-3s may reduce inflammation and block cytokine production, which interferes with lacrimal and salivary gland secretion.

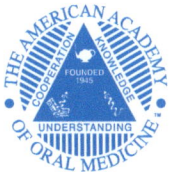

4 Complications of Dry Mouth

Etiology

Saliva is the principle protective bulk fluid for all oral tissues, which moisturizes and provides lubrication for hard and soft oral surfaces and is essential for speech, mastication, swallowing, taste, maintenance of general oral health and comfort. Without saliva, oral tissues become dry, friable and atrophic and may even crack (Table 6). Saliva as an integral part of the mucosal immune system, keeps bacterial and fungal populations under normal limits. Qualitative and quantitative loss of saliva, due to various diseases, disorders and side effects of active treatment, will negatively affect oral functions and efficiency.

TABLE 6: SIGNS AND SYMPTOMS OF DRY MOUTH
Sensation of dry/sore mouth
Multiple traumatic ulcers (cheek bite)
Enamel demineralization
Rampant dental carious lesion
Failures of dental restorations
Erythematous oral mucosa
Recurrent oral candidiasis
Difficulty in chewing and swallowing
Difficulty in speech
Intolerance to food spices and flavors
Recurrent sialadenitis
Retrograde infections

ORAL CANDIDIASIS

Saliva contains enzymes, immunoglobulins, and other molecules including lactoferrin, histatins and defensins that provide local antimicrobial activity. Quantitative and qualitative reduction of saliva can lead to decreased anti-microbial properties leading to clinical infection(s). The most common mucocutaneous fungal infection is Candida albicans (around 80%), although other can-didal species (e.g., Candida tropicalis, Candida krusei, or Candida glabrata) have been identified. Recurrent fungal infections occur in 30% to 70% of patients with Sjögren's syndrome, depending upon the disease activity and stage of the disease.

Clinical Description

Recurrent fungal infections are common in patients with dry mouth. A candidal infection may appear in one of four forms: erythematous candidiasis; pseudomembranous candidiasis (thrush); hyperplastic candidiasis and angular cheilitis. Erythematous candidiasis is more commonly associated with a dry mouth and appears as a red (erythematous) area most commonly on the palate or tongue (Figure 1A). The clinical appearance of pseudomembranous candidiasis is a white plaque that can be rubbed off with gauze (Figure 1B). Hyperplastic candidiasis appears as a white plaque that cannot be rubbed off. Angular cheilitis presents as redness and cracking at the corners of the mouth.

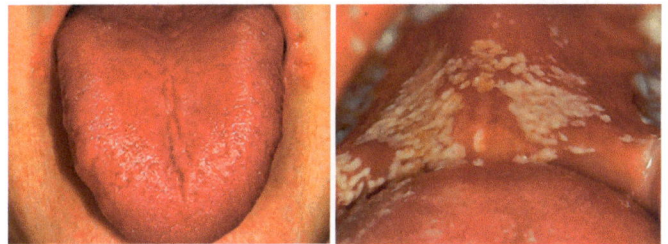

Figure 1A. *Erythematous candidiasis of the tongue*   Figure 1B. *Pseudomembranous candidiasis of the palate*

Diagnosis

The commensals can switch to pathogenic microorganisms with a favorable microenvironment in the oral cavity. The clinical appearance is often sufficient for a diagnosis of a fungal infection, and the start of appropriate anti-fungal therapy can be initiated. For refractory cases, culturing or biopsy of the lesion may be indicated.

Rationale for Treatment

Fungal lesions may cause pain, burning sensation and change in taste or if left untreated may lead to regional and systemic fungal infection. Therefore, appropriate anti-fungal therapy is indicated (Tables 7 & 8).

TABLE 7: GENERAL MANAGEMENT RECOMMENDATIONS FOR ORAL CANDIDIASIS
Topical (nystatin, clotrimazole, miconazole, amphotericin B)
Oral suspensions* Nystatin suspension Iatraconazole solution
Oral tablets (troche, pastille)* Clotrimazole (10mg) Miconazole (50 mg) buccal tablets Miconazole vaginal suppository used as an oral tablet *may be cariogenic from sucrose/glucose content*
Creams (for use with angular cheilitis)
Powders (for use with denture stomatitis – placed on tissue side of dentures)
Systemic (ketoconazole, fluconazole, itraconazole) Treatment of choice for more extensive oral fungal infections and if there is sufficient saliva to carry drug from blood stream to mouth. In severe salivary hypofunction, may be ineffective
Manual removal – brushing or scraping tongue

Treatment

Wearing dentures at night should be discouraged. Dentures hygiene should be maintained with brushing and denture cleansers, but in the case of candidiasis may be cleaned with a diluted chlorhexidine solution 0.12% overnight or a chlorhexidine gel 1% two times a day. The antifungal creams may be applied on the tissue side of the denture.

SALIVARY GLAND INFECTIONS
Etiology

Chronic salivary gland infections may occur in patients with dry mouth. The cause is often related to poor saliva drainage from the major salivary glands, which can lead to retrograde bacterial infections. Salivary stones (sialoliths) may form in glands and lead to enlargement of the parotid salivary gland or other major salivary glands. Salivary duct obstruction due to sialoliths is one of the main causes of sialadenitis. Acute bacterial parotitis most frequently occurs in older, debilitated patients, patients medicated with xerogenic drugs and/or patients with SS.

TABLE 8: MANAGEMENT OF ERYTHEMATOUS CANDIDIASIS
Treating of patients with "mild" to "moderate" candidiasis Nystatin suspension 100,000 IU/ml: Keep 5ml for 5 min in the mouth four-five times/day; spit or swallow for 7-14 days Clotrimazole (10mg) dissolve one troche five time a day for 7-14 days Miconazole (50 mg) buccal tablets daily for 7-14 days
In patients with visible salivary secretion and more extensive candidiasis Fluconazole tablets, 100 mg tablets: 2 tablets on the first day 1 tablet per day, for 1 to 4 weeks Weekly, monitor resolution of oral symptoms and signs Discontinue when both have resolved
Treating of patients with refractory candidiasis Select topical drug with lowest risk for dental caries Iatraconazole Solution 200mg 4X/day – swish and swallow Posiconazole suspension 400 mg 2X/day Voriconazole 200 mg 2X/day Oral or IV Amphotericin B 100mg/ml IV Echinocandins (Caspofungin, Micafungin, Anidulafungin) Continue drug until symptoms end and mucosal erythema resolves and filiform papillae return to dorsal tongue (4-10 weeks) If recurrence, retreat and consider maintenance dose of drug
For chronic suppression: Fluconazole 100mg three times a week.
For angular chelitis: Nystatin ointment Ketoconazole Clotrimazole Miconazole Also consider a combination of antifungal and antibacterial (e.g., nystatin and mupirocin) antifungals with steroids creams (e.g., nystatin/Triamcinolone, clotrimazole/betamethasone dipropionate, iodoquinol/hydrocortisons) to be applied at the corners of mouth for two/three times a day until the signs/symptoms are resolved.

The incidence is relatively low since antibiotics are so widely available and utilized. In any case, acute bacterial parotitis may be caused by a number of bacteria including, *Staphylococcus viridans*, *actinomycosis*, and *streptococci*. However, by far the most common organism is *Staphylococcus aureus*.

Clinical Description

An infected salivary gland is often noted by an enlargement of one or multiple major salivary glands (Figure 2). With an active bacterial infection, purulence can be expressed from the major salivary gland duct(s) (Figure 3). Increased swelling during salivary stimulation (e.g., during eating or chewing gum) is often reported with blockage of the salivary glands. Chronic major salivary gland swelling that does not change during salivary stimulation may appear with SS patients. For patients with parotid or submandibular gland enlargement or induration, but without symptoms or signs of acute bacterial

Figure 2: *Swelling of parotid gland due to retrograde infection in a patient with dry mouth.*

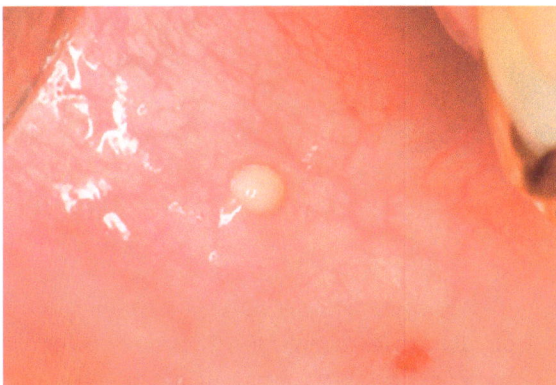

parotitis, it is prudent to first microscopically examine a smear of the exudate (e.g., with Wright stain or similar) to consider its cellular content, before prescribing antibiotics or to obtain a sample of the exudate for bacterial culture Similar appearing exudates to that seen in Figure 3 can also be seen in patients with SS, but contain only lymphocytes (i.e., no PMNs), and would not be appropriate for antibiotic therapy.

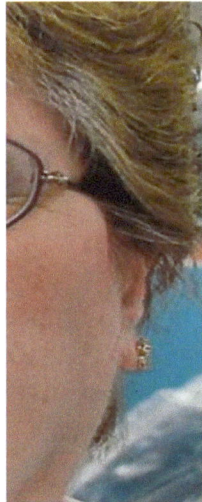

Figure 3: *Purulent drainage from an infected parotid gland.*

Enlarged glands in SS are most often a benign lymphoepithelial lesion (or lymphoepithelial sialadenitis), but close monitoring of these patients is important because the potential for progression to lymphoma.

Diagnosis

Aerobic and anaerobic culture and sensitivity testing of purulent discharge may be helpful to ensure appropriate antibiotic use. Interventional sialendoscopy is a new procedure for visualizing the salivary ducts. Progress in fiberoptic technology and miniaturization has allowed a rigid endoscope that is 1.3 mm in diameter and that has a working channel and several miniature wire baskets for retrieving small sialoliths using a sialendoscope in Stensen's or Wharton's duct. Small sialoliths can be extracted with the wire baskets whereas larger stones must first be fragmented.

These bacterial infections must be expeditiously diagnosed and aggressively treated with systemic antibiotics. Often the patients are debilitated, medically complex and may have multi-antibiotic resistance. Therefore, not only is swift and aggressive treatment with systemic antibiotics indicated but close follow-up and monitoring as well. Gram's stain and culture and sensitivity testing may be necessary.

Treatment

Intermittent swelling of the salivary glands without evidence of a bacterial infection can be treated with physical pressure to drain the gland. This will help remove accumulated debris in the ductal system. Other treatment options include the use of gustatory (sugar-free sour candies), masticatory (sugar-free gum) or pharmaceutical stimulation (i.e., cevimeline or pilocarpine) of the glands. An acute bacterial infection often necessitates the use of antibiotics such as Augmentin or Clindamycin.

Rx: Augmentin 500 mg capsules
Disp: 14
Sig: take one capsules qid po for one week

Rx: Clindamycin 150 mg tabs
Disp: 56
Sig: take two tabs qid po for one week

Rx: Dicloxacillin 500 mg tabs
Disp: 20
Sig: take one tab qid po for 5 days

Consideration for gland removal may be necessary for chronically enlarged glands that do not respond well to therapy and/or are an esthetic concern for the patient. The presence of sialoliths may necessitate gland removal or physical removal or ultrasound lithotripsy may help dislodge blockages of the ductal system. Gland removal should only be considered when other treatment options have been exhausted.

CARIES AND DENTAL EROSION
Introduction

The problems of caries and tooth wear are that each are multifactorial in presentation and etiology, caused by a complex interaction of physical, behavioral and environmental factors that make prediction of risk and prevention challenging. However, salivary gland function and saliva play a critical role in the processes that contribute to and prevent both problems with tooth integrity.

Saliva in a healthy, non-medicated and hydrated individual flows continuously and provides protection of the integrity and surface characteristics of the dentition by the following mechanisms:

1. Buffering of local acidic effects of cariogenic bacteria and extrinsic (e.g., dietary) and intrinsic (e.g., stomach acid) sources of acid that can chemically erode teeth;
2. Prevention of demineralization and promotion of remineralization of tooth surfaces promoted by the supersaturation of saliva with respect to calcium and phosphorus ions;
3. Antibacterial properties related to both immune and non-immune components of saliva, effecting virulence of cariogenic bacteria;
4. Influence on microbial colonization and biofilm formation on the teeth;
5. Aggregation and fluid clearance of cariogenic bacteria and other microbes by macromolecules in the saliva and role in swallowing function;
6. Viscosity created by mucins in saliva that lessen friction during mastication and soft tissue movement against the teeth;
7. Contribution to acquired pellicle of the tooth which provides a semi-permeable network of adsorbed macromolecules that partially protect against acidic attacks of tooth surfaces;
8. Increased salivary flow rate in response to acidic stimuli caused by refluxed stomach acids or ingested dietary acids, resulting in dilution and clearance of the acids.

The exact characteristics or components in saliva that contribute to caries or tooth wear initiation and progression are difficult to determine in humans due to multiple influences on salivary chemistry and flow rate, including the effects of time. However, the high frequency of damage to tooth structure evident when salivary function is compromised (especially flow rate) warrants careful assessment of risk factors for salivary gland dysfunction as part of routine workups for individuals with caries and tooth wear. It is only by identifying and managing these risk factors, alongside any needed restorative work, that the oral health care provider can help the patient attain a sustainably healthy and intact dentition.

Caries

Caries is the most common pathological condition in children in the United States, caused primarily by poor oral hygiene with plaque retention of acid-producing mutans *Streptococci* and *lactobacilli* and frequent fermentable carbohydrate dietary intake, combined with lack of access to regular preventive care. New caries occurrence and recurrence extend into adulthood and elder years, with salivary dysfunction and periodontal disease (causing gingival recession exposing root surfaces) playing a larger role. Declining cognitive and sensory ability and decreasing manual dexterity make it difficult to maintain adequate self-care in advanced years of age. Poverty and disabling medical conditions which lead to unemployment increase lack of access to professional care and increase risk of caries. Lack of education about healthy eating habits or lack of money or access to healthy foods also contribute to the caries problem. Untreated caries may lead to tooth loss, decreased ability to eat healthy foods, decrease in systemic health and decrease in quality of life.

Importance of Caries Risk Assessment

It is now recognized that detection and repair of tooth structure damaged by caries itself is not sufficient to manage the caries disease process. Additionally, not all carious lesions need to be managed surgically. Accurate diagnosis of arrested caries or shallow sub-surface caries that are reversible with chemotherapeutic management can prevent placement of a restoration that itself can become a risk factor in the presence of an oral environment that promotes caries. Risk factors for caries must be identified and addressed to prevent caries development and recurrence. Prevention of caries is critically important, since restorative and prosthodontic dental care may be out of reach for the most vulnerable populations where caries rates are the highest. Therefore, caries risk assessment should be included in all basic dental examinations.

Salivary Function and Caries

In the caries balance schema described by Featherstone (2003), low salivary flow and impaired salivary gland function play a prominent role in development of caries created by acidic challenges to teeth by cariogenic bacteria. The main causes of impaired salivary function in adults are side effects of medications used to treat various medical conditions, substance abuse, autoimmune disease such as Sjögren's syndrome and radiation treatment that includes the head and neck region. Individuals who have these conditions have very high risks of caries, as well as oral mucosal disease, due to the decrease in protective effects provided by saliva. Therefore, it is critical to assess and manage salivary dysfunction when treating caries infection regardless of the cause of the dysfunction.

Correspondingly, adequate salivary flow and its protective components (described earlier) offer a counterbalance to caries-creating forces. It is equally important to improve salivary function as much as possible to allow natural defense mechanisms provided by saliva to protect tooth integrity. These steps should augment other tooth protective strategies such as topical fluorides and remineralizing agents, antibacterial agents, adequate oral hygiene procedures and non-cariogenic dietary habits.

Basics of Caries Risk Assessment

Caries risk assessment forms available online from organizations such as the ADA and the Journal of the California Dental Association can assist the provider in determining caries risk, which will help guide preventive treatment. The version for individuals above 6 years of age are more pertinent for patients with salivary dysfunction.

The presence of active caries or history of caries or tooth loss due to caries in the previous 3 years remain the strongest predictors of new caries, but other risk factors play a role. Risk factors that can be identified during problem and medical history-taking include any conditions that impact salivary flow rate, such as medication side effects, autoimmune disease (e.g., Sjögren's syndrome), radiation therapy affecting the head and neck region, eating disorders and substance abuse. Questions about saliva that correlate with low salivary flow rate include self-assessment of the amount of saliva or history of difficulty swallowing, dryness while eating, and/or needing sips of water to swallow dry food.

Special health care needs that limit adequate oral hygiene also increase caries risk. Specific questions about lifetime exposure to fluoride via drinking water, supplements, toothpastes or professional application, access to regular professional dental care, frequency of intake of sugary foods or drinks or, in the case of a child, caries experience of the mother, caregiver or siblings, can inform the provider of contributing conditions to caries risk.

Risk factors that are identified during clinical examination include presence of active caries by visual inspection or radiographs, missing teeth due to caries, heavy plaque, deep pits or fissures in tooth anatomy, presence of interproximal restorations, fixed or removable prosthodontic or orthodontic appliances, defective restorations, and exposed root surfaces. Signs of low salivary flow besides caries, such as dryness and atrophy of the mucosal tissues, candidiasis, fissured tongue and oral malodor, are evidence of salivary dysfunction and increased caries risk.

It is recommended that measuring flow rate of whole resting and stimulated saliva be performed to assess salivary function (See Chapter 2) A flow rate of less than 0.1 ml/min for resting whole saliva and less than 1.0 ml/min for stimulated whole saliva indicates increased risk for caries.

Other biological risk factors for caries are high concentrations of caries-producing bacteria (mutans *streptococci* and *lactobacillus*) in the saliva, which reflect bacterial levels in plaque. Several commercial kits are available to measure bacteria by culture-based methods such as the Caries Risk Test by Vivadent and Dentocult by GC America.

Caries Treatment and Risk Reduction

The caries risk assessment tools assign a low, medium, high or extremely high-risk rating for caries. Once a patient's level of caries risk is determined, individualized preventive measures can be designed to manage the risk. Patients with caries and very low salivary flow, indicated either by clinical appearance of oral tissues or by salivary flow measurements, are considered high risk for caries. Clinical guidelines for caries management for patients with low salivary flow and high risk of caries, regardless of cause, are listed in Table 9 on the following page.

Tooth Erosion and Other Forms of Tooth Wear

Loss of tooth surface that is not caused by caries is one of the most under-diagnosed and misdiagnosed of tooth problems due to its insidious nature. Erosion of tooth surfaces by acids not caused by bacteria is particularly easy to miss if one is not familiar with its early signs or if one is not alert for erosion when medical or dietary risk factors are present in an individual. A common error in diagnosis is to interpret occlusal and cuspal loss of

TABLE 9: CLINICAL GUIDELINES FOR CARIES MANAGEMENT IN HIGH RISK PATIENTS WITH SALIVARY HYPOFUNCTION (STIMULATED WHOLE SALIVA FLOW RATE <1 ML/MIN)		
GOAL: Detect Caries Early and Monitor Risks[‡]		
Key Steps	• Caries Bacteria Test	Test for determining mutans Streptococci and Lactobacilli counts in saliva, conduct initially and at every recall visit to assess efficacy and patient cooperation.[* ‡]
	• Salivary Flow Test	Measure flow rates for resting and unstimulated whole saliva, initially and at every recall visit to assess efficacy and patient cooperation.[** ‡]
	• Bitewing Radiographs	Every 6 months – Until no cavitated lesions are evident [‡]
	• Recall Examinations	Every 3-4 months to evaluate for caries, patient education and fluoride varnish application.
GOAL: Reduce Plaque Levels/Acidity		
Key Steps	• Oral Hygiene Instruction	Recommend sonic toothbrush, if possible, for more effective plaque removal. Interdental cleaning with floss or brushes are also advised. Brush tongue
	• Diet Analysis and Guidance	Record dietary intake for 4 days. Assess frequency of fermentable carbohydrates and acidic foods and beverages. Provide dietary guidelines for reduction as needed.
	• Neutralizing Rinses	Baking soda rinses or chewing gum with baking soda, 4–6 times daily (Home recipe: 2 tsps. of baking soda in an 8 oz. bottle of water)
GOAL: Increase Salivary Flow		
Key Steps	• Adequate Hydration	Drink approximately 8 glasses of water daily, urine should be colorless or light yellow.
	• Stimulation of Salivary Flow	Xylitol chewing gum or lozenges (6–10 grams/day) two tabs of gum or lozenge 4 times daily. Use adhesive xylitol containing tablets at night. Use other sugarless and/or acid neutralizing gums or lozenges if xylitol gum is not accessible.
	• For Medication –induced Salivary Gland Dysfunction	Physician Consult – Consider change in medication dosage, timing, formulation and/or type, change in number of medications.
	• For Autoimmune Disease-related or Radiation-induced Salivary Hypo-function	Rx Sialogogues (if salivary glands are able to secrete saliva): Pilocarpine, 5-10 mg, three times daily, for at least 3 months to assess efficacy Cevimeline, 30 mg, three times daily, for at least 3 months to assess efficacy
GOAL: Protect/Restore Tooth Integrity		
Key Steps	• Home Fluoride Application	1.1 % NaF toothpaste twice daily– Rx toothpaste or 0.2% NaF Rinse daily, one bottle (Rx), followed by OTC 0.05 % NaF rinse twice daily or when mouth feels dry or after snacking or meals or 0.454% Stannous fluoride toothpaste twice daily (has antibacterial properties in addition to enamel protection properties.)
	• Professional Fluoride Application	5 % NaF varnish on all teeth, 1–3 applications initially, every recall exam
	• Sealants	Resin-based or fluoride-releasing glass-ionomer for teeth with susceptible pits and fissures
	• Treatment of Cavitated Lesions	Composites or resin-based or fluoride-releasing glass ionomer restorations for active, cavitated carious lesions Eradication of carious lesions ASAP Silver Diamine Fluoride (38%) Use to arrest caries in patients who cannot tolerate restorative care or who must be stabilized so they can be restored over time or patients with little or no access to definitive restorative care.
	• Diet Modification	Advise eating cheese (if no contraindications exist) after an acidic challenge to the teeth to help remineralize tooth surfaces. Milk closely resembles saliva.

enamel, in the form of pits into the cusps exposing dentin, as caused solely by bruxism. This leads to incomplete or incorrect treatment consisting only of providing a patient an occlusal guard, when in fact, diet modification or medical management of GERD to reduce acid exposure of the teeth may also be necessary.

TABLE 9: CLINICAL GUIDELINES FOR CARIES MANAGEMENT IN HIGH RISK PATIENTS WITH SALIVARY HYPOFUNCTION (STIMULATED WHOLE SALIVA FLOW RATE < 1 ML/MIN) *(CONTINUED)*		
GOAL: Reduce Carious Bacteria		
Key Steps	• Antibacterial Rinse	Chlorhexidine gluconate (0.12 %) rinse – 10 ml rinse for one minute daily for one week each month, used one hour before fluoride toothpaste use
	• Xylitol Chewing Gum or Lozenge	Xylitol chewing gum or lozenge (6–10 grams/day- approximately two tabs of gum or lozenge) 4 times daily

Adapted from: Jenson L, Budenz AW, Featherstone JDB, Ramos-Gomez F, Spolsky VW, Young D. Clinical Protocols for Caries Management by Risk Assessment. *J Calif Dent Assoc* 2007; 35:714-723.
‡ Recommendations for frequency of monitoring caries risk after baseline assessment by caries bacteria tests, salivary flow rate assessment and radiographs may change as more clinical trials are conducted. *e.g., Caries Risk Test (CRT) marketed by Vivadent, (Amherst, NY). Dentocult by GC America
**eg. Saliva-Check BUFFER by GC America

Since early erosive wear of the teeth is asymptomatic, it is usually noticed by the astute oral health care provider during visual examination of the teeth before the patient notices it. Careful evaluation of medical history, medication use, substance use, habits, diet and review of systems (e.g., for symptoms of GERD) is critical. Physical assessment includes documentation of the degree of loss by photos or models. Salivary functional assessment is important to assess flow rate and buffer capacity, since saliva plays a role in protecting against acidic challenges, regardless of the source.

Multifactorial Etiology of Tooth Wear

It is extremely important to realize that tooth wear seldom has a single cause. In addition to multiple possible sources of excessive acid exposure (e.g., stomach acids or dietary excess), there can often be other contributors to tooth wear in each person, including occlusal or incisal attrition due to a bruxism habit or cervical or facial enamel abrasion from aggressive oral hygiene habits, exacerbated by salivary dysfunction. Incomplete management of all causes of tooth wear will result in progression of tooth surface loss, potentially leading to an extensively damaged dentition requiring complex care.

Recognizing and considering risk factors for all types of tooth wear during history-taking can assist the provider in obtaining a thorough diagnosis and management plan. Table 10 on the following page shows the characteristics, risk factors, evaluation and treatment of erosion, attrition and abrasion side by side.

Dental Restorative Material for Dry Mouth

Restorative therapies to manage caries in those with salivary dysfunction should be conservative and minimally invasive. For initial treatment, subgingival margins and full coronal coverage should be avoided whenever possible as these areas are most susceptible to recurrent decay and are less accessible to cleansing, antimicrobial and remineralization strategies. Full veneer crowns, if necessary, should not be placed until caries is under complete control. Vital pulp therapy using stepwise remineralization and biocompatible dental materials to allow smaller restorations or maintenance of existing complex restorations should be considered.

Silver amalgam has the advantage of being technique insensitive, with self-sealing margins and excellent wear resistance. A fluoride releasing amalgam has been developed, but the amount of fluoride released was small and of short duration. Amalgam bonding agents enable conservative restoration but are sensitive to conditions where isolation and hemorrhage control may be less than ideal.

Fluoride releasing composite resins release little long-term fluoride, unlike resin modified glass ionomers. The use of direct restorative materials such as composites, glass ionomers, copomers and giomers tend to be technique sensitive and require proper material selection based on occlusal load, size of restoration, and location of restoration and secondary caries risk.

Conventional and resin modified glass ionomers are able to release fluoride and are "rechargeable" in that they are able to act as a reservoir, taking-up and releasing fluoride available in the oral environment. There is an array of glass ionomers available with different properties and differing abilities to recharge and release fluoride into the oral environment. For a posterior restoration, the stronger glass ionomers with higher liquid to powder ratios may be used, but there is a reduced capacity for fluoride release and recharge. Specific issues have arisen regarding the use of these restoratives in persons with salivary dysfunction:

TABLE 10: ASSESSMENT AND MANAGEMENT OF THE PATIENT WITH TOOTH WEAR						
	EROSIVE WEAR				**ATTRITION**	**ABRASION**
Etiology GASTRO-ESOPHAGEAL REFLUX DISORDER/ VOMITING	Intrinsic Factors	Extrinsic Factors	Contributing Factors		BRUXISM/ PARAFUNCTION	TOOTH-BRUSHING HABITS/tooth contact with abrasive substances or objects
	DIETARY ACIDS/ OCCUPATIONAL EXPOSURE	SALIVARY HYPOFUNC-TION	HISTORY OF ALCOHOLISM			
1. GATHER HISTORICAL INFORMATION Identify medical and dental risk factors and their symptoms from the history.	• obesity • family history of Gastro-Esophageal Reflux Disorder (GERD) • history of hiatal hernia • taking proton pump inhibitors, H2 blockers, OTC antacids • pregnant state • alcoholism • medication side effect (nausea or vomiting) • eating disorder (bulimia) • preoccupation with food or exercise • medications for depression **Symptoms:** • heartburn • gastric pain • history of hoarseness • sense of something stuck in throat • difficulty swallowing • acid taste in mouth • excessive burping • nausea • excessive salivation • night awakening with excessive coughing	• high level of consumption of acidic beverages or foods • prolonged and/or frequent contact of teeth with acidic medications or supplements (eg. Vitamin C chewable tables) **Occupational Exposure:** • professional wine tasting • competition level swim training in non-pH controlled pool water • exposure to acidic fumes in the work environment **Symptoms:** • tooth hypersensitivity (uncommon unless individual is child or adolescent or erosion advances rapidly)	• medication side effect (salivary hypofunction) • taking 1 or more medications • autoimmune disease such as Sjögren's syndrome • family history of autoimmune disease • diabetes, poor glycemic control • history of head and neck or total body radiation treatment for cancer **Symptoms:** • difficulty eating and swallowing • sense of too little saliva • oral mucosal disease (e.g., candidiasis)	Increased risk for: • GERD • vomiting • salivary hypofunction • high intake of acidic alcohol-containing drinks **Risk Factors for Alcoholism:** • Family history of alcoholism or substance abuse • Depression • Anxiety • Schizophrenia **Definition of Alcohol Abuse:** • >15 drinks / week if male. • >12 drinks / week if female. • >5 drinks /day at least once a week (binge drinking)a	• awareness of parafunction **Risk Factors for TMD** (Temporomandibular Disorder): • family history of TMD • history of: teeth grinding and clenching, inability to open or close jaw completely, tension-type headaches, preexisting pain conditions (e.g., low back, genital, fibromyalgia) • irritable bowel syndrome • poor sleep quality, sleep disruption **Symptoms:** • masticatory muscle fatigue or tightness • TMJ locking, • jaw, neck or face pain or soreness • increased tooth pain or sensitivity • pain simulating an earache, ringing in the ears	• older age • use of a hard-bristled toothbrush • history of brushing in a horizontally back and forth manner across the teeth excessively and/ or with an abrasive dentifrice • chewing betel nut or abrasive foods or friction from non-foods (dust) • using teeth to bite or hold items • history of smoking cigarettes (contributes to gingival recession, exposure of root surfaces) **Symptoms:** • tooth hypersensitivity (not common)

Table 10 continues on next page →

TABLE 10: ASSESSMENT AND MANAGEMENT OF THE PATIENT WITH TOOTH WEAR *(continued)*						
EROSIVE WEAR					**ATTRITION**	**ABRASION**
Etiology GASTRO-ESOPHAGEAL REFLUX DISORDER/ VOMITING	**Intrinsic Factors**	**Extrinsic Factors**	**Contributing Factors**		**BRUXISM/ PARAFUNCTION**	**TOOTH-BRUSHING HABITS/tooth contact with abrasive substances or objects**
	DIETARY ACIDS/ OCCUPATIONAL EXPOSURE	**SALIVARY HYPOFUNCTION**	**HISTORY OF ALCOHOLISM**			
2. PHYSICAL EXAMINATION / Recognize typical appearance of various types of tooth wear.	• "cupping" of cusp tips with or without dentin exposure • loss of tooth surface in • non-occluding areas • chipping of weakened incisal edges	• loss of enamel from palatal surfaces of anterior teeth secondary to GERD, excessive vomiting	• enamel may be intact at the gingival crest area • smooth, shallow wear • facial surfaces of anterior teeth may exhibit loss of surface characteristics	• Occlusal cuspal pits and significant amount of exposed dentin on occlusal surface • tooth wears away faster than adjacent dental restoration	• matching occlusal wear of opposing teeth with even wear of dentin and enamel • teeth are flattened, loose, fractured, chipped	• often called Non-Carious Cervical Lesions (NCCL's) • may be broad and shallow or deep and wedge-shaped at the cervical areas of teeth • first premolar teeth commonly affected • exposed cementum due to gingival recession
Recognize appearance of tooth wear with multi-factorial etiology	**Erosion and attrition** Smooth facial enamel erosion with incisal edge thinning or chipping, due to high intake of acidic beverages to moisten dry mouth Flattened matching wear of opposing incisal and occlusal surfaces of teeth from attrition due to bruxism.		**Erosion from high intake of dietary acid and frequent vomiting secondary to alcohol abuse** Loss of facial surface characteristics, posterior teeth with cuspal pits and exposed dentin in a 27-year-old female with weekend alcohol binge drinking.		**Erosion, attrition and abrasion** Shallow, broad cervical erosive wear in 34-year-old male due to intake of several cans of pineapple juice daily for 2 years, aggressive tooth-brushing and bruxism habit.	**Erosion and abrasion** Wedge-shaped cervical lesions in 31-year-old male with GERD and aggressive horizontal brushing technique.

Table 10 continues on next page ➡

		GERD	BULIMIA	SALIVARY DYS-FUNCTION	ALCOHOL ABUSE	SIGNS OF BRUXISM HABIT	NOTE on the term "ABFRACTION"
2. PHYSICAL EXAMINATION	Look for other physical signs indicating presence of medical or behavioral risk factors for tooth wear.	• oropharyngeal area may be inflamed in appearance • excessive amounts of saliva • obesity • halitosis • hoarseness • intermittent voice loss • wheezing • signs of smoking habit (nicotinic stomatitis)	• non-inflammatory enlargement of parotid glands (sialoadenosis) • facial puffiness • bloodshot eyes dry, blotchy skin • hoarseness • dry, cracked lips • inflammation or ulcers of the oral mucosa • scars, calluses or teeth marks on the knuckles or fingers caused by self-induced vomiting • weight fluctuations	• inability to express saliva from salivary gland orifices • foamy saliva • lack of salivary pooling in the floor of the mouth • dry, sticky mucosa, atrophic mucosa • fissuring of tongue • decreased papillation of the tongue	• non-inflammatory enlargement of parotid glands (sialoadenosis) • decreased salivary function • mucosal inflammation • spider angiomas on face • jaundice • flushed appearance • decrease in attention to personal hygiene	• hypertrophy of masseter muscles • crenulations on lateral surface of the tongue • linea alba of the buccal mucosa • increased tooth pain or cold sensitivity • joint or masticatory muscle palpation pain, • limited or abnormal jaw opening • TMJ noise with opening/closing with pain or limitation • Moderate to severe malocclusion	• describes the result of tensile and compressive forces during tooth flexure causing fatigue wear at the dental cervical area with resultant microfractures • limited evidence that abfraction causes wedge-shaped defects at the cervical areas of teeth • may lead to undue emphasis on occlusal equilibration for treatment of tooth wear

TABLE 10: ASSESSMENT AND MANAGEMENT OF THE PATIENT WITH TOOTH WEAR (continued)

Document and monitor all types, amount and location of tooth wear with models or intraoral photographs.

- Moisture is needed for optimal bonding and setting of these restoratives. The lack of saliva could affect the ultimate performance of these materials.
- If a patient has these types of restorations, then neutral fluoride is preferred as the acidic nature of some fluoride solutions could erode the surface of the glass ionomer.
- The manufacturer recommends the placement of an unfilled resin over the finished restoration. The selection of this resin is critical and some of these resins can reduce movement of the fluoride ion between the tooth and the oral cavity.

Copomers are the newest group of fluoride releasing materials that are light cured and similar to composite resins in their handling characteristics. Their fluoride release and recharge rates are lower than glass ionomers and are unproven in patients with high caries rate secondary to salivary hypofunction.

A giomer is a direct restorative material that is pre-charged with fluoride during manufacture and is rechargeable in association with high levels of intraoral fluoride. There is the added advertised benefit of a local ability to neutralize acid, to inhibit biofilm formation and to disrupt the mature biofilm by release of ions including sodium, strontium aluminum silicate and borate. There is extremely limited research on the additional bioactive features of this material in the dry mouth.

Dental implants have been successfully placed in individuals with Sjögren's syndrome, although the literature supporting their use is scarce. A careful pre-surgical assessment is important with attention to immunosuppression status, the use of immunosuppressants and biphosphonates, and the ability to keep the implant area clean.

BURNING MOUTH
Etiology
Oral burning is a common complaint in dry mouth patients. Many local or systemic conditions may be the underlying cause, which may be from tissue trauma from decreased saliva lubrication, candidiasis, habit, iron deficiency, vitamin B_{12} deficiency, uncontrolled diabetes, central neuropathy (i.e.,

Parkinson's disorder), peripheral neuropathy (i.e., acoustic neuroma) and contact sensitivity/allergy. There have also been reports of burning pain associated with use of angio-tensin-converting enzyme (ACE) inhibitors. Burning mouth syndrome (BMS) is a neuropathic pain condition character-ized by a burning pain in the oral and perioral tissues. Epide-miological surveys have reported a prevalence rate for BMS between 0.7% and 2.6%, with an NIH survey estimating close to 1 million burning mouth sufferers in America. Although most prevalent amongst postmenopausal women, men and women of any age can also be affected. Other sensory changes commonly associated with BMS include dysgeusia, dysesthesia and perceived xerostomia. These possibilities should be ruled out prior to a diagnosis of BMS.

The cause of BMS is still under discussion, however most specialists agree that the sensations are related to a neu-ropathy. One model suggests that damage to one of the taste nerves (CN VII, CN IX) disrupts the co-inhibitory rela-tionship between these pathways and the oral pain path-ways (CN V). As a result of this loss of inhibition, the pain pathway exhibit over-excitability and abnormal output.

Clinical Description

Burning pain symptoms can can impact any tissue surface, depending on the underlying etiology (Figure 4). BMS can involve one or multiple sites and commonly reported areas include the upper and lower lips, tip of the tongue, dorsal surface of the tongue, palate and throat. The pain is com-monly present bilaterally, but may also be unilateral. The pattern of pain and sensory changes throughout the day are described as minimal on waking and increase through-out the day to a maximum in early afternoon and night. Most patients report the sensations remit on eating and

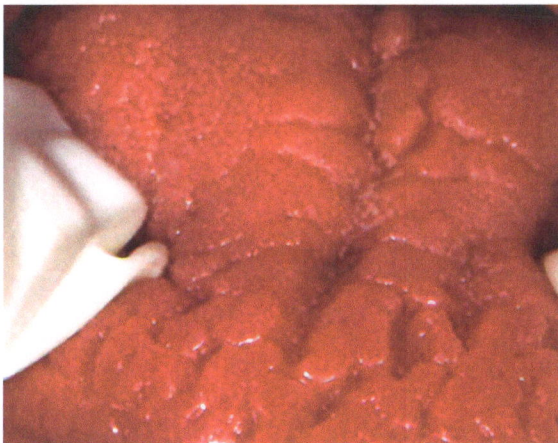

Figure 4: *Friable burning mucosa causes severe pain, discomfort and loss of function*

are not disruptive to sleep. The BMS symptoms are usually present daily.

There are usually no changes to the mucosa with BMS but BMS can co-present with local tissue changes. The changes that have been observed may include geographic tongue, lichen planus and candidiasis infection. Addressing these tissue changes usually will not resolve the burning of BMS symptoms.

Other sensory changes associated with BMS include taste changes, gagging, coughing and dysesthesia, including described sensations of 'sandiness,' 'roughness,' 'dryness,' and "sensitivity." The patients may report dry mouth despite evidence of normal salivary output. Taste changes are common, including both taste loss and phantom taste sensations. Phantom sensations of a bitter, metallic or foul taste may be reported. These other sensory changes related to BMS may be just as or more disturbing than the burning pain and the multitude of symptoms add to the difficulty in diagnosing BMS.

Diagnosis

Clinical tests which may be helpful to rule out another cause to the burning pain include:

- Hematological tests for: CBC, glucose, nutritional factors, autoimmune panel including ANA, anti-SSA
- Oral cultures for fungal, viral or bacterial if suspected
- MRI to rule out central changes, especially if pain is unilateral, atypical or does not respond to medication
- Salivary flows for unstimulated and stimulated whole saliva (<1.5 ml/15min, unstimulated; <4.5 ml/15 min stimulated)
- Salivary uptake scan may be considered if low salivary flows and Sjögren's syndrome suspected
- Allergy testing, if needed, especially to dental panel of allergens
- Removal of possible offending medications including ACE inhibitors

Rationale for Treatment

Depending on the underlying etiology, appropriate treat-ment to control conditions such as hematinic deficiencies, diabetes, neuropathies, salivary hypofunction and aller-gies will alleviate burning symptoms. The most effective treatment for BMS, like many neuropathic pain disorders, appears to be the use of anticonvulsant medication. Topi-cal rinses and ointments may also used with some success. Some BMS cases will remit spontaneously with time and the rationale for BMS treatment is to control the disruptive pain and sensations until remission.

Treatment

TOPICAL MEDICATION:

Successful use of benzodiazepines in a rinse for topical use has been reported. Other topical formulations containing capsaicin have been reported in small trials to be helpful for BMS also.

Rx: Capsaicin cream 0.025%
Disp: 1 tube
Sig: Apply sparingly to affected sites qid. Wash hands after each use and keep away from eyes. May cause temporary exacerbation of symptoms.

SYSTEMIC MEDICATION:

There is literature supporting the use of GABA-acting anticonvulsants such as benzodiazepines with good results. A very low dose is usually sufficient, and several agents can be used in combination in order to reduce the adverse effects of these medications; the most commonly reported being drowsiness and dizziness.

Rx: Clonazepam (0.25 - 0.5mg)
Disp: 0.5mg
Sig: Start with ½ tab before bed and titrate up to 1 tab before bed as needed.

If this is not effective or only partially effective:

Rx: Gabapentin (100-1800mg)
Disp: 100mg
Sig: Start with 1 cap during time of the day the pain is worst and titrate up a maximum of 3 caps tid as needed. Increase dosage slowly by 100mg per day.

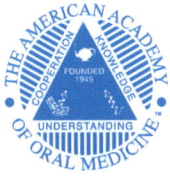

5   Sjögren's Syndrome

Etiology

Women make up 90% of patients with Sjögren's syndrome. The average age at onset is about 50 years, but the age range is wide and includes a small number of children. Sjögren's syndrome is considered the second most common connective tissue autoimmune disease affecting up to 3.1 million Americans or approximately 1 in 70 persons. This number doubles when including those with another major autoimmune disease and symptoms of Sjögren's syndrome. The underlying cause of Sjögren's syndrome is unknown.

Clinical Description

Decreased saliva production and qualitative changes in the saliva and oral flora characterize Sjögren's syndrome. The signs and symptoms from salivary gland dysfunction are discussed in more detail in Chapter 4. Early in its course, most patients complain of symptoms of dry mouth (xerostomia), while others may complain of difficulty chewing or swallowing food, difficulty wearing a lower denture, or oral burning symptoms (which are usually associated with chronic candidiasis–discussed in Chapter 4–or due to mucosal friction from poor lubrication related to salivary hypofunction). The onset of these symptoms is usually insidious. However, some patients with significant signs of salivary dysfunction do not complain of oral symptoms.

The clinical signs of salivary dysfunction in Sjögren's syndrome include a reduced or absent salivary pool in the floor of mouth, reduced mucosal lubrication, and a pattern of progressive dental caries (located in cervical areas, incisal edges of anterior teeth, or cusp tips of posterior teeth). Thickened or cloudy-appearing saliva may be expressible from the parotid or submandibular ducts. About one third of patients develop signs of chronic erythematous candidiasis (i.e., loss of filiform papillae from the dorsal tongue and bilaterally symmetrical areas of mucosal erythema, with or without angular cheilitis).

TABLE 11: SYSTEMIC OR INTERNAL ORGAN MANIFESTATIONS WITH SJÖGREN'S SYNDROME
General: fatigue, malaise, fevers
Ear, nose, and throat: epistaxis, otitis media, conduction deafness, recurrent sinusitis
Gastrointestinal: esophageal dysmotility, esophageal webs, reflux, atrophic gastritis, autoimmune pancreatitis, liver disease
Genitourinary: vaginitis sicca, interstitial cystitis
Hematologic: anemia, leukopenia, lymphopenia, cryoglobulinemia, lymphoma
Lungs: xerotrachea, recurrent bronchitis/pneumonia, lymphocytic interstitial pneumonitis, pulmonary fibrosis, bronchiectasis, bronchiolitis obliterans, BOOP*
Neurologic: peripheral neuropathy, cranial neuropathy, central nervous system involvement
Renal: interstitial nephritis, hyposthenuria, renal tubular acidosis (types 1, 2)
Rheumatologic: arthralgias, polyarthritis, myalgias, myositis, Raynaud's phenomenon
Skin: xeroderma, purpura, urticaria, vasculitis
BOOP - bronchiolitis obliterans and organizing pneumonia

Approximately 20-30% of patients experience prolonged bilateral enlargement of the parotid or submandibular glands, which are firm (but not hard) and non-tender to palpation. When examined by biopsy, these tumors are usually diagnosed as lymphoepithelial lesion (or lymphoepithelial sialadenitis), which is a benign reactive process. However, these chronic tumors may transform into MALT (mucosa-associated lymphoid tissue) lymphomas, which are usually indolent for many years, but later can give rise to a rapidly growing high-grade lymphoma. Non-Hodgkin's B-cell lymphomas occur in 3-4% of individuals with Sjögren's syndrome.

About 20-30% of affected individuals develop one or more systemic or internal organ manifestations (Table 11). Internal organ manifestations can also be the presenting manifestations of the disease and may precede the onset of clinically significant xerostomia in 20% of cases. Morbidity of the internal organs in Sjögren's syndrome occurs as a consequence of exocrine gland dysfunction and/or lymphocytic invasion. The internal organ manifestations of those with Sjögren's syndrome and other autoimmune disease such as rheumatoid arthritis or systemic lupus erythematosus reflect that of the underlying connective tissue disease and are, therefore, not included in the present discussion.

Diagnosis

When a patient has the symptoms or clinical signs described above and is not taking drugs or have past medical treatment that would likely cause the symptoms, Sjögren's syndrome must be considered. Because of the probability that other organ systems may be involved, the dentist should consult with the patient's physician and the patient should be referred to an ophthalmologist to examine for keratoconjunctivitis sicca (KCS). There is no single test that will diagnose Sjögren's syndrome, or other related autoimmune syndromes. The current classification criteria for Sjögren's syndrome, known as the American College of Rheumatology/European League Against Rheumatism (ACR/EULAR) classification criteria for Sjögren's syndrome, are summarized in Table 12 on the next page.

The most disease specific assessment of the salivary component of American College of Rheumatology/ European League Against Rheumatism classification criteria for Sjögren's syndrome is from a labial salivary gland (LSG) biopsy. This office procedure consists of local anesthetic infiltration, a 1.5–2.0 cm incision just through normal appearing lower lip mucosal epithelium, careful dissection of 4 or 5 minor salivary glands, one at a time, from the subepithelial connective tissue and closure, as necessary, with resorbable sutures. A LSG biopsy is not always necessary for symptomatic patients who have objective evidence of the oral and ocular components of Sjögren's syndrome associated with the serum marker autoantibodies anti-Ro (a.k.a. anti-SSA). However, patients with KCS and signs of salivary dysfunction who lack serum anti-Ro/La, would need a LSG biopsy exhibiting focal lymphocytic sialadenitis and a focus score ≥ 1 focus/4 mm^2 to diagnose Sjögren's syndrome.

Salivary function is most easily assessed by measuring whole unstimulated salivary flow for 15 minutes (see Chapter 2). Functional assessments of salivary flow can quantify patients' salivary production as a severity measure or can be used to assess disease progress over time. Various means of imaging salivary glands (e.g., contrast sialography, magnetic resonance, ultrasound or combinations of those) have been proposed to diagnose the salivary component of Sjögren's syndrome, but do not assess function and are not yet sufficiently disease specific to replace LSG biopsy.

Rationale for treatment

Sjögren's syndrome is a chronic, autoimmune rheumatic disease characterized by lymphocytic infiltration of exocrine glands. The most common symptoms include dry mouth, dry eyes (keratoconjunctivitis sicca), fatigue and musculoskeletal pain. The glandular manifestations of dry mouth and dry eyes and the multitude of extraglandular manifestations can have a significant impact on quality of life.

Treatment

Treatment regimens for the signs and symptoms of dry mouth are discussed in sections 3, which include topical comfort agents as well as masticatory, gustatory, and pharmacologic stimulants.

Rituximab (anti-CD20), is FDA-approved for treatment of rheumatoid arthritis, targets B cell proliferation, and may improve the extraglandular manifestations, dry eyes and dry mouth complaints. Only weak evidence supports the use of Rituximab as a possible therapeutic consideration for xerostomia in Sjögren's syndrome where there is some evidence of residual salivary function and significant evidence of oral damage as determined by the clinician, and for whom conventional therapies, including topical moisturizers and secretagogues have proven insufficient. Further randomized trials are needed. TNF-alpha inhibitors should not be used to treat the dry eye and dry mouth symptoms of individuals with Sjögren's syndrome unless there are also symptoms of rheumatoid arthritis or associated conditions. Additional biological therapies are currently in the pipeline for the management of Sjögren's syndrome and will not be discussed in this monograph.

TABLE 12: AMERICAN COLLEGE OF RHEUMATOLOGY/EUROPEAN LEAGUE AGAINST RHEUMATISM (ACR-EULAR) CLASSIFICATION CRITERIA FOR PRIMARY SJÖGREN'S SYNDROME:

The classification of primary Sjögren's syndrome applies to any individual who meets the inclusion criteria,[a] does not have any of the conditions listed as exclusion criteria,[b] and has a score of ≥4 when the weights from the 5 criteria below are summed.

Item	Weight/score
Labial salivary gland with focal lymphocytic sialadenitis and focus score of ≥ 1 foci/4 mm[2c]	3
Anti-SSA/Ro positive	3
Ocular Staining Score ≥5 (or van Bijsterveld score ≥4) in at least 1 eye[d,e]	1
Schirmer's test ≤ 5mm/5 minutes in at least 1 eye[d]	1
Unstimulated whole saliva flow rate ≤ 0.1 ml/minute[d, f]	1

[a] These inclusion criteria are applicable to any patient with at least 1 symptom of ocular or oral dryness, defined as a positive response to at least 1 of the following questions: 1) Have you had daily, persistent, troublesome dry eyes for more than 3 months? 2) Do you have a recurrent sensation of sand or gravel in the eyes? 3) Do you use tear substitutes more than 3 times a day? 4) Have you had a daily feeling of dry mouth for more than 3 months? 5) Do you frequently drink liquids to aid in swallowing dry food?, or in whom there is a suspicion of Sjögren's syndrome (SS) from the European League Against Rheumatism SS Disease Activity Index questionnaire (at least 1 domain with a positive item).

[b] Exclusion criteria include prior diagnosis of any of the following conditions, which would exclude diagnosis of SS and participation in SS studies or therapeutic trials because of overlapping clinical features or interference with criteria tests: 1) history of head and neck radiation treatment, 2) active hepatitis C infection (with confirmation by polymerase chain reaction, 3) AIDS, 4) sarcoidosis, 5) amyloidosis, 6) graft-versus-host disease,) IgG4-related disease.

[c] The histopathologic examination should be performed by a pathologist with expertise in the diagnosis of focal lymphocytic sialadenitis and focus score count, using the protocal described by Daniels et al.

[d] Patients who are normally taking anticholinergic drugs should be evaluated for objective signs of salivary hypofunction and ocular dryness after a sufficient interval without these medications in order for these components to be a valid measure of oral and ocular dryness.

[e] Ocular staining score described by Whitcher et al; van Bijsterveld score described by van Bijsterveld.

[f] Unstimulated whole saliva flow rate measurement described by Navazesh and Kumar

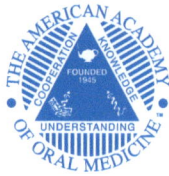

6 Hypersalivation

Etiology

The sensation of excessive secretion of saliva may be due to an increase in saliva production (true hypersalivation) or a decrease in salivary clearance (sialorrhea or ptyalism). True hypersalivation is uncommon, but can be caused by medications, numerous neurological conditions and certain heavy metals (Table 13). Other causes are gastroesophageal reflux disease, hyperhydration, the secretory phase of menstruation and organophosphorous (acetylcholinesterase) poisoning. A less productive hypersalivation may result from nausea, infant teething or local irritations, such as aphthous ulcers or an ill-fitting oral prosthesis. Sialorrhea is usually associated with swallowing difficulties or compromise of the circumoral musculature.

TABLE 13: CAUSES OF HYPERSALIVATION
Direct Cholinergic/muscarinic agonists   Bethanechol, Pilocarpine, Arecoline, Cevimeline

Indirect Cholinergic/muscarinic agonists
    Edrophonium, Neostigmine, Physostigmine,
    Pyridostigmine, Metrifonate, Donepezil, Galantamine,
    Rivastigmine, Tacrine

Other salivary stimulating medications   Lithium, Clozapine, Risperidone, Nitrazepam

Neurological conditions
    Parkinson's disease, Wilson's disease, Amyotrophic
    lateral sclerosis, Down syndrome, Fragile X syndrome,
    Autism, Cerebral vascular accident (CVA), Myasthenia
    gravis, Cerebral Palsy, Facial paralysis, Guillain-Barré
    syndrome, Moebius syndrome, Congenital suprabulbar
    palsy, Hydrocephalus, Freeman-Sheldon syndrome,
    Psychosis, Brain tumors, Seizures, Worster-Drought
    syndrome, Landau-Kleffner syndrome, Encephalitis,
    Angleman syndrome

Exposure to heavy metals   Iron, Lead, Arsenic, Mercury

Clinical Description

Hypersalivation can result in drooling, with the concurrent clinical effects of perioral dermatitis, cheilitis and fungal infections. In severe cases, a partial or total blockage of the airway, which can lead to aspiration of oral contents and aspiration pneumonia. Psychosocial issues can occur due to social embarrassment and rejection.

Diagnosis

It is essential to obtain an exact history of the hypersalivation as well as a complete past and current medical history. A systematic oral evaluation should be performed. Since most cases of hypersalivation are actually a secretion clearance issue, a swallowing study should be obtained from a clinician with expertise in speech and swallowing. A salivary flow rate should be obtained. Collection of unstimulated whole saliva that results in more than 1 ml/min suggests greater than normal production of saliva and can help differentiate between an over production of saliva versus a salivary clearance issue.

Exposure to heavy metals (Iron, Lead, Arsenic, Mercury), can be a cause of hypersalivation, particularly in children. The source of the exposure can include environmental contamination, an improperly processed water supply, industrial waste, and hobbies. A complete history of the patient's work and living habits can help identify the potential heavy metal source. If suspected, urinalysis, a complete blood count, including a peripheral smear and a tissue examination (particularly hair and nails) should be obtained.

Premenopausal women should be evaluated for potential pregnancy, and in postmenopausal or male patients, androgen levels should be determined to rule out an androgen-secreting tumor. If the onset is acute, a CT of the brain should be obtained to rule out a CVA or a central nervous system mass.

Rationale for Treatment

Hypersalivation treatment should take into consideration the etiology of the hypersalivation, the risk versus benefit of the treatment, and most importantly, the quality of life of the patient.

Treatment

Depending on the etiology, there are three types of treatments for hypersalivation: physical therapy, medications, and surgery.

PHYSICAL THERAPY:

Physical therapy can be used to improve neuromuscular control, but patient cooperation is essential. Speech and swallowing therapy should be attempted prior to medical or surgical interventions. Unfortunately, studies have shown a low success rate with this therapeutic modality.

DRUG-BASED TREATMENTS:

Drug treatments for hypersalivation are devised based upon etiology. If the patient is experiencing hypersalivation secondary to a pharmaceutical treatment, alternate medications can be evaluated, and if the therapeutic profile cannot be altered, compatible xerostomic agents (see below) should be considered. Consultations should be made with the patient's physician to help prevent deleterious drug-drug interaction problems or polypharmacy-induced side effects. Hypersalivation that occurs secondary to chronic nausea (e.g., during chemotherapy) can be treated with antiemetic medications. Hypersalivation due to gastroesophageal reflux disorder (GERD) is a protective buffering response to acids encountered in the oral cavity. The GERD should be treated and under most circumstances, the hypersalivation will resolve. If a diagnosis of heavy metal toxicity has been made, patient will need to be treated with chelating agents. Neurological and neuromuscular conditions (e.g., CVA, Down syndrome, central neurological infections) can result in neuromuscular incompetence in swallowing function, resulting in salivary pooling in the anterior floor of the mouth and salivary spillage from the oral cavity (drooling). The most common cause of drooling in children over the age of 4 is Cerebral Palsy and in adults, it is Parkinson's disease.

Intraglandular injections of botulinum toxin have been used to decrease salivary flow. There is no standard as to the number of units that are to be given in the treatment of hypersalivation. For botulinum toxin A, a number of 1U/kg can be used with relative safety. In adults, there is variability in the literature as to the dosage, which ranges from 40U/gland to 100U/gland. As with all botulinum toxin injections, the response is only temporary and necessitates re-infiltration 2-4 months later. The most common complications are thickening of the saliva and a temporary dysphagia. Ultrasound guidance has been found to increase accuracy with the injection.

SURGICALLY-BASED TREATMENTS:

There are a multitude of surgical techniques that have been devised to treat hypersalivation. Historically, redirection of the submandibular ducts and parotid ducts posteriorly to the tonsillar pillars has been performed, although patients with poor salivary clearance will not benefit from this technique. Bilateral tympanic neuronectomy has also been performed, but this leaves a permanent anesthesia to the anterior portion of the tongue and is not recommended. Another surgical technique is bilateral submandibular gland excision with parotid duct ligation or just ligation of all four major salivary gland ducts. These techniques are successful in reduction of drooling approximately 80% of the time. The advantage of the four-duct ligation technique is that it involves an intraoral surgical approach, thereby reducing the risk of damaging the facial nerve.

MEDICATIONS:

> **Rx**: Scopolamine
> Disp: 1.5mg Transdermal Patch
> Sig: Place patch on hairless area
> *Transdermal scopolamine lasts for 3 days and has been successful in the management of hypersalivation, but it is contraindicated in smaller children.*

> **Rx**: Propantheline
> Disp: 15mg tablets
> Sig: 1 tablet PO tid to qid

> **Rx**: Benztropine
> Disp: 0.5 to 2mg tablets
> Sig: *The usual daily dose is 1-2 mg, with a range of 0.5 to 6 mg orally. Generally, older patients, and thin patients cannot tolerate large doses. Patients with behavioral and psychological disorders are usually poor candidates for therapy.*

Rx: Atropine
Disp: 0.4mg tablets
Sig: 1 po qd-tid

Rx: Glycopyrrolate
Disp: 1mg tablets
Sig: 1 po qd-tid
  *Glycopyrrolate tablets are not recommended for
  use in pediatric patients under the age of 12 years.*

Rx: Diphenhydramine Hydrochloride (Benadryl)
Disp: 25mg-50mg
Sig: Take 25–50mg 3–4 times daily as needed

The above-referenced drugs are anticholinergic medications used to decrease saliva production. Side effects of anticholinergic drugs include: tachycardia, arrhythmia, blurred vision, photophobia, dryness of the eyes/nose/throat, nausea, constipation, urinary retention, somnolence, hallucinations (visual or aural), mental disorders, dry warm skin, flushed skin, oral lesions, and dermatitis. Drugs with anticholinergic activity, such as phenothiazines and tricyclic antidepressants, can increase anticholinergic effects when used concurrently.

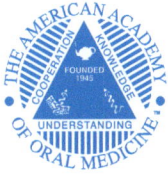

7 Halitosis

Prevalence and Etiology

Halitosis is a common presenting complaint among dental patients. Although, for most patients, this diagnosis and its treatment can be straightforward, for many others a patient complaint of bad breath can prove to be challenging and complex to treat. According to one recent systematic review of over five hundred published articles on halitosis, the average worldwide prevalence was shown to be almost 32%, a rate suggesting a trend towards increasing. Halitosis can be classified into categories of genuine halitosis, pseudo-halitosis, and halitophobia. Genuine halitosis is diagnosed if obvious malodor with intensity beyond socially acceptable level is perceived. If obvious malodor is not perceived by others, although the patient stubbornly complains of its existence, it is diagnosed as pseudo-halitosis. Should a patient, after treating either genuine or pseudo-halitosis resulting in no objectively noticeable foul odor, still believe that he or she has halitosis, very likely the diagnosis is halitophobia. Genuine halitosis could be either physiologic or pathologic.

Physiologic halitosis, also termed transient halitosis, is temporary and occurs when volatile odoriferous hematologically-borne substances are liberated into the lungs from food, such as herbs, spices, and some vegetables such as onion, garlic, and cabbage. Another type of physiologic halitosis is morning breath. This condition most likely results from stagnation of epithelial cells and food debris, increased microbial metabolic activity during sleep that is aggravated by a physiological reduction in salivary flow, lack of nocturnal physiologic oral cleansing (e.g., movement of the facial and oral muscles) and variable oral hygiene procedures prior to sleep. Hunger and starvation can also lead to a similar malodor. Habits such as smoking tobacco or drinking alcohol, can also lead to transient bad breath.

Pathologic halitosis arises by the same mechanisms as the physiologic type plus the pulmonary release of blood-borne substances. This type is distinct in quality, more intense, persistent and not easily reversible originating from regional or systemic pathoses that require treatment of the underlying disease. In more than 85% of people suffering from bad breath, the etiology is localized to the oral cavity and is mostly produced by the action of gram negative anaerobic bacteria on sulfur-containing proteinaceous substrates such as cystine and methionine in the saliva, debris and plaque. The primary molecules responsible for oral malodor are the microbial degradation products, volatile sulfur compounds (VSC) such as hydrogen sulfide (H_2S), methyl mercaptan (CH_3SH) and dimethyl sulfide (CH_3SCH). Oral inflammatory processes resulting in ulceration and tissue necrosis may also harbor the gram-negative bacteria and lead to bad breath. Non-oral regional causes of oral malodor include chronic sinusitis, tonsillitis and the presence of tonsilloliths. The remaining 15% may indicate an underlying systemic disease. Among such conditions are liver cirrhosis and hepatic failure, uremia associated with kidney failure, ketoacidosis in diabetes mellitus, gastric *Helicobacter pylori* infections and dyspepsia, pyloric stenosis and trimethylaminuria.

Halitophobia, also known as imaginary halitosis, is a phenomenon seen in individuals who complain of halitosis that cannot be detected by others. Some of these patients may become depressed and the belief may become so profound that it dominates their lives, and even lead to the thought of suicide. It is an "olfactory reference syndrome", which is a recognized psychiatric condition, where the patient has an olfactory delusion that they emit a foul smell from the mouth or elsewhere. These patients need referral to mental health professionals for management.

Diagnosis

The evaluation of a patient with a complaint of bad breath consists of an adequate history to identify all the local and systemic factors that may be related to the bad breath complaint, a complete examination and an analytical or sensory (organoleptic) evaluation of patient's breath.

The examination involves a thorough physical evaluation of the head and neck structures, and intraoral examination of the dentition, periodontal tissues, various oral mucosal sites and the salivary glands. This assessment is necessary to determine if patient has tooth decay, broken restorations, malpositioned teeth and partial impactions that can make oral hygiene difficult and periodontal disease. Radiographic examination of the dentition should also be included. Several health centers also include an endoscopic sinus examination as part of their routine patient evaluation.

The organoleptic method is the examiner's perception of a subject's oral malodor. This is the most practical clinical procedure for evaluating a patient's level of oral malodor. Patients should be instructed to abstain from ingesting any food, chewing and drinking, usual oral hygiene practices, using oral rinses and breath fresheners and smoking for 2 hours before the assessment. Patients are also instructed to avoid using scented cosmetics for 24 hours before the assessment, to abstain from eating garlic, onion and spicy foods for 48 hours and to abstain from taking antibiotics for 2 weeks before the assessment. Organoleptic measurement can be carried out by the sniff test (smelling the patient's expired breath) and the tongue odor (smelling the scrapings from the dorsal surface obtained with a plastic spoon). After smelling these samples, oral malodor is rated on a 5-point scale (detection threshold 0 and maximum detection 5). For reliable diagnosis, the oral malodor assessment should preferably be carried out by two or three independent odor judges.

The analytical methods of assessing VSCs are either in-vitro salivary-based tests or in-vivo assessment of the exhaled air. One example of a salivary-based test is benzoyl-DL-arginine-naphthylamide (BANA) test that is based on the enzymatic activity of gram-negative bacteria; the incubated saliva sample is analyzed to determine the bacterial strains involved. The in-vivo assessment of the expired air may be accomplished by employing gas chromatography (GC) or by using portable VSC sensors. GC is considered the most accurate test for measuring oral malodor because of its specificity for volatile sulfur compounds but it requires specialized expensive equipment and skilled technicians to conduct the test. A number of portable VSC sensors are available for clinical use, unfortunately when measured against GC and organoleptic methods, their accuracy in diagnosing halitosis is not consistent. The earliest portable sensor introduced into the marketplace in early 1990's was Halimeter® (Interscan Corporation, USA) that tests the total sulfur-containing compounds (mostly hydrogen sulfide) in a fixed volume of expired air. Since then, other sensors that have become available include Breathtron® (New Cosmos Electric, Japan) that uses a zinc-oxide semiconductor technology to detect VSCs, Breath Alert™ (Tanita Corporation, Japan) a portable sulfide monitor and OralChroma™ (Abilit Corporation, Japan) a portable GC device. In clinical practice, these sensors may be more useful in monitoring treatment efficacy over time than for diagnosing halitosis. In essence, the organoleptic testing is the gold standard for diagnosing halitosis.

Rationale for Treatment

Oral malodor can have a significant psychological impact on a patient and confirmation by available subjective and objective diagnostic tests will guide the clinician to appropriate management strategies.

Treatment

The results of a complete oral soft tissue examination, evaluation of the dentition and the periodontal tissues determine the course of malodor treatment. When a systemic condition is suspected, patients should be referred for medical evaluation and treatment. Patients with pseudo-halitosis or halitophobia should be counseled appropriately and referred for psychological evaluation and treatment.

All faulty restorations, active decay or dental pulp pathology or other oral disease must be appropriately diagnosed and treated. In the absence of any specific oral pathology, the origin of physiological halitosis is mainly the presence of excessive tongue coating. Gentle mechanical cleaning of the dorsal aspect of the tongue and the use of chemical disinfecting mouth rinses along with the daily oral hygiene routines are used for oral malodor management. Mouthwashes containing chlorite anion and chlorine dioxide have been shown to be effective in oxidizing and inactivating the oral VSCs, demonstrating long lasting effects. Chlorhexidine rinses, especially with cetyl pyridium chloride or zinc, have also been shown to significantly reduce the microbial load of the tongue and saliva. Finally, in small studies, a number of natural remedies have started to show promising results in reducing the VSC levels in-vitro and in patients with halitosis. Some examples are: Ayurvedic antimicrobial compounds such as Mimusops elengi (Spanish Cherry), other natural antimicrobials such as champignon extract, green tea extract, and essential oils such as tea tree oil and cinnamon bark. Larger clinical trials are needed to show if any of the natural remedies can produce long-lasting effects in the treatment of

halitosis. It should also be noted that thus far, the use of probiotics has only produced modest clinical improvement in oral malodor but not in measurable reduction of VSCs.

Table 14 summarizes the treatment strategies for oral malodor:

TABLE 14: TREATMENT STRATEGIES FOR ORAL MALODOR	
General Recommendations	*Specific Recommendations*

- Management of faulty restorations, active decay or dental pulp pathology and periodontal disease
- Management of oral soft tissue conditions
- Avoid odiferous foods like onions, garlic, cabbage, radishes, cauliflower
- Avoid tobacco and alcohol use
- Reduce the consumption of red meat and dairy products
- Avoid staying hungry
  ▸ Eat healthy snacks between meals
- Practice good oral hygiene
  ▸ Home care including brushing, flossing, denture care
  ▸ Regular professional cleaning
- Maintain moisture in the mouth
  ▸ Adequate hydration
  ▸ Sugarless gum
	- Tongue scraping on a daily basis
	- Use commercial antibacterial mouthwashes
	  ▸ Chlorine dioxide, cetyl pyridinuim chloride, phenolic flavor oil, zinc chloride, triclosan, chlorhexidine and other rinses
	- Saliva substitutes or sialogogues if xerostomia present
	- Use nasal irrigation if post nasal drip present
	- Refer for ENT evaluation of chronic sinusitis/post nasal drip, tonsillitis, tonsillolith
	- Refer for medical evaluation of systemic conditions

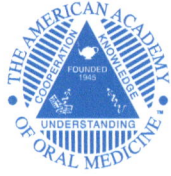

8 Chemosensory Disorders

The actual prevalence of chemosensory disorders is unknown. Recent estimates of the prevalence of self-reported chemosensory alterations from the 2011-2012 US National Health and Nutrition Examination Survey (NHANES) are 23% for smell and 19% for taste alterations. About 90% of chemosensory disorders are chronic and 40% of them occur in those over the age of 65. Taste and smell are essential sensory systems for nutrition food selection, and for detection of imminent danger such as gas leaks, or smoke. Distorted, diminished or loss of chemosensation can significantly deteriorate one's quality of life. Chemosensory disorders affect in particular a disproportionately large segment of the elderly population. Taste disorders cannot be discussed in the absence of smell disorders which are much more frequent among patients. The vast majority of patients who complain of a taste loss or diminished taste in reality suffer from olfactory loss. Only 1 out of 10 patients who think they have a taste disorder turn out to have one (Table 15).

TABLE 15: Percent of Patients Who Subjectively Think They Either Have Smell and/or Taste Loss, and % of Patients After Diagnosis Who Turn Out to Have That Diagnosis.		
Complaint	% of subjective complaint	% with the correct diagnosis
Smell and taste loss	57	2.5
Smell loss only	20	60
Taste loss only	10	0.9

OLFACTORY DISORDERS
Etiology
The sense of smell involves the ability to detect and identify odors. For olfaction to occur optimally, the nasal airway should be patent, the nasal mucosa should be healthy and coated with sufficient viscous mucous, and the neural pathways responsible for olfaction should be intact. Smell disorders are more common than taste losses due to slow turnover of olfactory neurons (30-60 days) and the distinct innervation of the olfactory system. In contrast, taste cells have a more rapid turnover (10-20 days) as well as present bilaterally and have multiple innervation involvement. The location of olfactory receptors high in the nasal cavity makes them susceptible to variability in nasal patency and airflow patterns that potentially limit access of odorants. Also, the position of olfactory nerve axons near the cribriform plate makes them vulnerable to tearing or severing from forces associated with head injury.

Etiologic factors associated with olfactory disorders are either related to transport dysfunction (odorants cannot make contact with functioning olfactory neoroepithelium) or sensorineural dysfunction (odorants cannot be processed due to neural injury or damage). These include:

- Sinonasal conditions, such as allergic rhinitis, chronic rhinosinusitis and nasal polyps
- Nasal and paranasal sinus disease
- Upper respiratory tract infections
- Head and facial trauma
- Sinonasal neoplasms
- Environmental toxins
- Medications
- Aging
- Chronic medical conditions, such as endocrine diseases and cancer
- Neurodegenerative disorders, including Alzheimer's disease, Parkinson's disease, and Multiple Sclerosis
- Psychiatric conditions
- Congenital disorders (e.g., Kallman syndrome)
- Surgical procedures (e.g., middle ear surgery)
- Idiopathic

Clinical Description

Smell dysfunction can have the following clinical presentations:

- Anosmia – complete loss of smell
- Hyposmia – partial loss of smell
- Dysosmia – alteration or distortion of smell, which can be further categorized as:
  - Parosmia / Troposmia - perception of an odor (usually unpleasant), triggered by a stimulus
  - Phantosmia – perception of an odor without a stimulus present (olfactory hallucination)

The majority of flavor perception is derived from odorants. Thus, many patients who present with a complaint of flavor or taste loss in actuality have smell loss, and require olfactory assessment.

Diagnosis

- Medical and dental history – documentation and differentiation of the specific chemosensory abnormality (smell, taste, or both).
- Physical examination – including thorough otolaryngologic and neurologic assessments. Referral to a multidisciplinary taste and smell center may be useful when diagnosis of the specific disorder cannot be readily established.
- Chemosensory tests
  - Commercially available psychophysical odor discrimination tests such as the University of Pennsylvania Smell Identification Test (UPSIT), Brief Smell Identification Tests and Burghart Sniffin' Sticks determine a patient's ability to identify a series of common odorants (e.g., coffee, pizza, chocolate, lilac).
  - Odor detection threshold tests utilize progressively stronger concentrations of an odorant such as butanol or phenyl ethyl alcohol to determine the weakest dilution that a patient can detect. Each nostril must be tested separately to determine if the smell disturbance is unilateral or bilateral.
  - Trigeminal function for the common chemical sense is assessed by a patient's ability to detect a pungent odor such as menthol.

- Imaging: Computed tomography, magnetic resonance imaging, positron emission tomography and single photon emission tomography are useful for ruling out intracranial or peripheral nerve abnormalities.
- Laboratory tests may be necessary to diagnose underlying medical abnormalities.

Rationale for Treatment

Olfactory dysfunction can impact a patient's quality of life, and decreased or abnormal olfactory ability can increase a patient's risk for toxic exposures (e.g., natural gas, smoke, poisons, spoiled food). Olfactory loss has also been associated with dementia, mild cognitive impairment (MCI), and Alzheimer's disease. Standardized tests of odor identification are widely available, and may be a useful tool to improve diagnostic and predictive accuracy for cognitive decline, neurodegenerative disorders and mortality in older adults.

Treatment

Treatment is highly dependent upon the specific etiologic factor. Olfactory disorders will sometimes resolve spontaneously in the absence of any treatment (Table 16).

TABLE 16: MANAGEMENT STRATEGIES FOR OLFACTORY DISORDERS
Pharmacotherapy
• Systemic & topically applied intranasal corticosteroids for reducing mucosal edema and shrinking nasal polyps
• Antibiotics, decongestants and antihistamines for chemosensory losses due to bacterial sinus infection and allergic rhinitis
• Benzodiazepines, tricyclic antidepressants and anticonvulsants may also be helpful for patients with dysosmias. Some examples are: ‣ clonazepam 0.5–2 mg hs   ‣ amitriptyline 25–100 mg hs   ‣ gabapentin 300–2000 mg per day
Surgery
• Endoscopic and nasal sinus surgery for obstructive disorders may result in return of normal olfactory function if more conservative approaches are unsuccessful
Miscellaneous
• Treatment should include counseling on smoke and natural gas detection, and labeling of food to track spoilage
• Baseline and repeat chemosensory testing are useful in assessing prognosis for recovery of normal function
• Patients should be informed that recovery of olfactory function may take several years or may never occur, particularly following post-viral infection or head trauma

TASTE DISORDERS
Etiology

It is estimated that up to 15% of Americans might have taste and/or smell disorders but do not seek help. Patients often confuse taste and smell disorders. Up to 1.1 million Americans suffer from diagnosable taste disorders. Among the most common causes of taste disorders are infections of bacterial, viral or fungal origin. Another common cause

TABLE 17: FREQUENTLY PRESCRIBED MEDICATIONS OR ORAL PRODUCTS AND THEIR EFFECT ON TASTE.		
Class of Drugs	**Medication**	**Symptom**
Anesthetics	benzocaine, lidocaine	ageusia
Antidiabetic	biguanide	metallic dysgeusia
Antineoplastic	bleomycine, 5-fluorouracil, methotrexate	bitter or sour dysgeusia
Antithyroid agents	methylthiouracyl	ageusia
Cardiovascular	diltiazem, nifedipine	hypogeusia, dysgeusia
Muscle relaxant	baclofen	ageusia, hypogeusia
Oral products	sodium lauryl sulfate	sweet or salty ageusia

for taste disorders is medications such as antibiotics, antihypertensives, anticonvulsants, antiproliferatives, antiinflammatories, lipid-lowering medications, angiotensin-converting enzyme inhibitors (ACE inhibitors), antiparkinson, antihistamines and antiretrovirals (Table 17).

Anesthesia or surgery-induced injuries to the cranial nerves that supply the gustatory system are a frequent iatrogenic cause of taste disorders. Such procedures include mandibular block, extraction of wisdom teeth, tonsillectomy or surgery of the middle ear. Patients complain of phantom, metallic, bitter or salty tastes on the side of the surgery, usually noticeable within hours after the anesthesia wears off. The loss may be temporary or permanent. Injury to the Chorda tympani may also appear secondary to viral or bacterial infections such as chronic otitis media, Bell's palsy or Ramsay Hunt Syndrome.

Smoking may have an adverse affect on taste sensitivity and discrimination. Similarly, radiation to the oral region may lead to mucositis, xerostomia and impaired taste sensation. Aging has only a moderate effect on taste, with sour and bitter tastes being most affected. Finally, patients wearing dentures, where a significant portion of the oral mucosa is covered, are deprived of some gustatory, thermal and somatosensory sensations.

Clinical Description

The specific terms used for taste disorders are ageusia (lack of taste), dysgeusia (abnormal taste or phantom taste), hypogeusia (reduced taste), and hypergeusia (increased sense of taste). All of the above disorders can be generalized, partial or specific to a particular taste quality. The most common complaint is of an unusual taste in their mouth. This may occur in the absence of any stimulus, or when eating a particular food. Patients may also complain

of metallic, bitter, sour, or salty tastes, but rarely of sweet taste. In some instances, patients will complain of reduced sense of taste, lack of flavor, lack of enjoyment of food, or a loss of the usual taste associated with their favorite food. Complete loss of taste is very rare. Loss of taste in a specific area of the tongue, in particular following a surgical or dental procedure, is usually restricted to one side, and typically to the area of innervation of the Chorda tympani branch of the facial nerve. Those involving the glossopharyngeal or the vagus nerves are less frequent.

Diagnosis

Whenever a patient is tested for taste functions, they should also be tested for olfactory functions, a more likely and about 9 times more frequent source of complaint. First, a detailed medical and dental history is compiled followed by a physical examination. Several tests are available to identify taste disorders, some of them suitable in a non-specialized clinical setting (Table 18 on next page).

TOPICAL ANESTHESIA:
To identify if dysgeusia or phantom taste is local or central in origin one can administer a simple test with the use of topical and local anesthesia. Topical anesthesia can be applied to a small area if a complaint is localized; or to the whole mouth, if the complaint is generalized. Apply a small amount of unflavored 1% dyclonine hydrochloride or 2% viscous lidocaine hydrochloride to the tongue with a cotton swab. For the whole mouth test, the patient is asked to keep 5 mL of 0.5% dyclonine and 0.5% dyphenhydramine in 0.9% saline in the mouth for one minute, expectorate, rest another minute and rinse with water. (Note: it is important to warn patients about the danger of aspiration due to a reduced gag reflex following anesthesia.) During testing the patient is asked to describe the quality and intensity of the taste complaint (usually dysgeusia

TABLE 18: CHAIR-SIDE DIAGNOSIS OF FREQUENT TASTE DISORDERS			
Complaints	**Finding**	**Possible Diagnosis**	**Treatment**
Sudden loss of taste following mandibular block, extraction of wisdom teeth	Restricted to one-side, anterior 2/3 of the tongue	Injured Chorda tympani	No treatment, spontaneous resolution may occur
Sudden loss of taste	Restricted to one-side, anterior 2/3 of the tongue including facial asymmetry	Bell's Palsy	No treatment, spontaneous resolution may occur
Gradual generalized diminished sense of taste	Subjective complaint, no objective finding. Patient complains of "food does not taste as it used to"	Olfactory loss, upper respiratory infection, obstruction, head trauma	Specialized diagnosis and treatment
Gradual or sudden appearance of unusual taste sensation (metallic, bitter, salty, sour)	Subjective complaint, often no objective finding	Side effect of medications, drug metabolites in saliva	Remove, substitute medication. Effect may linger for months.
Gradual or sudden appearance of unusual taste sensation (bitter, foul taste)	Oral and perioral infections White plaque on the tongue	Poor oral hygiene Candida albicans, immunocompromised patient, HIV	Institute rigorous oral hygiene, resolve oral infections, anti-retroviral treatment

or phantom taste). If the complaint diminishes or disappears, then the cause is probably local. If anesthesia does not eliminate the taste complaint, then the cause could be olfactory related, or central, and the patient should be referred to a specialist.

MANDIBULAR BLOCK ANESTHESIA:

Similar to topical anesthesia, dysgeusia and phantom taste can also be diagnosed by administration of the mandibular block. This form of anesthesia affects both the trigeminal and the Chorda tympani nerve but not the glossopharyngeal nerve. Such selectivity is not possible with topical anesthesia. During the mandibular block, patients are questioned about the status of their complaint. A reduction in the complaint may indicate a local problem. If the complaint persists the source is probably not peripheral and the patient should be referred to a specialist.

Additional diagnostic methods exist, but they exceed the expertise of non-specialized clinics. These diagnostic tests include detection threshold, spatial taste testing, magnitude matching, and the use of the electrogustometer.

Rationale for Treatment

Taste dysfunction can significantly impact a patient's nutrition and quality of life.

Treatment

There are no effective ways of treating taste disorders. Treatment is highly dependent on diagnosis (Table 18). Where a local etiology is identified (e.g., infections, medications) appropriate treatment can be instituted. Interestingly, there is a considerable body of literature covering the use of zinc in the treatment of taste disorder. This treatment still remains controversial. No extensive double-blind study has convincingly demonstrated the efficacy of this medication. Therefore, zinc should not be prescribed as a blanket treatment. Some taste disorders may resolve even in the absence of any intervention. In a retrospective study of 48 patients, two thirds of the patients experienced spontaneous resolution of dysgeusia within 10 months.

THIS PAGE INTENTIONALLY
LEFT BLANK

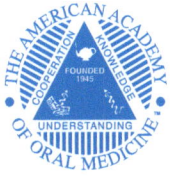

References

- American Dental Association Caries Risk Form (Age >6) (http://www.ada.org/~/media/ADA/Science%20and%20Research/Files/topic_caries_over6.ashx)

- Brignardello-Petersen R. 2017. "A new mouthwash with low concentrations of chlorhexidine seems to reduce intraoral halitosis and volatile sulfur compounds in patients after 12 hours of use." *J Am Dent Assoc* 148(4):e6. doi: 10.1016/j.adaj.2016.11.030. PubMed PMID: 28193474.

- Bromley SM, Doty RL. 2010. "Olfaction in dentistry." *Oral Dis.* 16(3):221-32. doi: 10.1111/j.1601-0825.2009.01616.x. PubMed PMID: 19732354.

- Burgess JO and Gallo JR. 2002. "Treating root surface caries." *Dent Clin N Am* 46:385-404.

- Burt BA. 2006. "The use of sorbitol- and xylitol-sweetened chewing gum in caries control." *J Am Dent Assoc* 137:190-196.

- California Dental Association Caries Risk Form (Age. 6) (https://www.cda.org/Portals/0/journal/journal_102007.pdf)

- Carsons SE, Vivino FB, Parke A, Carteron N, Sankar V, Brasington R, et al. 2017. "Treatment Guidelines for Rheumatologic Manifestations of Sjögren's Syndrome: Use of Biologic Agents, Management of Fatigue, and Inflammatory Musculoskeletal Pain." *Arthritis Care Res* (Hoboken). 69(4):517-27. doi: 10.1002/acr.22968. PubMed PMID: 27390247.

- Cummins MJ, Papas A, Kammer GM, Fox PC. 2003. "Treatment of primary Sjögren's syndrome with low-dose human interferon alfa administered by the oromucosal route: combined phase III results." *Arthritis Rheum* 49:585-93.

- Daniels T. 1984 "Labial salivary gland biopsy in Sjögren's syndrome. Assessment as a diagnostic criterion in 362 cases." *Arthritis Rheumatol* 27:147-56.

- Daniels TE, Cox D, Shiboski CH, Schiodt M, Wu A, Lanfranchi H, et al. 2011. "Associations between salivary gland histopathologic diagnoses and phenotypic features of Sjögren's syndrome among 1,726 registry participants." *Arthritis Rheum.* 63(7):2021-30. doi: 10.1002/art.30381. PubMed PMID: 21480190; PubMed Central PMCID: PMCPMC3128201.

- Dawes C. 2004. "How much saliva is enough for avoidance of xerostomia?" *Caries Res* 38:236-240.

- Dawes C, Pedersen AML, Villa A, Ekstro J, Proctor GB, Vissink A, Aframian D, McGowan R, Aliko A, Narayana N, Sia YW, Joshi RK, Jensen SB, Kerr AR, Wolff A. 2015. "The functions of human saliva: A review sponsored by the World Workshop on Oral Medicine VI" *Arch of Oral Biol* 60: 863–874.

- Devanand DP. 2016. "Olfactory Identification Deficits, Cognitive Decline, and Dementia in Older Adults." *Am J Geriatr Psychiatry*" 24(12):1151-7. doi: 10.1016/j.jagp.2016.08.010. PubMed PMID: 27745824; PubMed Central PMCID: PMCPMC5136312.

- Diagnosis and Management of Dental Caries Throughout Life, National Institutes of Health, 2001. Bethesda, Md.

- Do T, Damé-Teixeira N, Naginyte M, Marsh PD. 2017. "Root Surface Biofilms and Caries." *Monogr Oral Sci* 26:26-34.

- Drug Information Handbook for Dentistry. 22 ed. 2016. Alphen aan den Rijn, The Netherlands: Wolters Kluwer

- Epstein JB, van der Meij EH, Lunn R, Stevenson-Moore P. 1996. "Effects of compliance with fluoride gel application on caries and caries risk in patients after radiation therapy for head and neck cancer." *Oral Surg Oral Med Oral Pathol Oral Radiol Endod* 82:268-275.

- Featherstone JDB. 2003. "The caries balance: Contributing factors and early detection." *J Calif Dent Assoc* 31:129-133.

- Featherstone JDB, Domejean-Orliaguet S, et al. 2007. "Caries risk assessment in practice for age 6 through adult." *J Calif Dent Assoc* 35:703-7,710-3.

- Featherstone JDB, Singh S, Curtis DA. 2011. "Caries Risk Assessment and Management for the Prosthodontic Patient." *J Prosthodont* 20:2-9.

- Foulks GN, Forstot SL, Donshik PC, Forstot JZ, Goldstein MH, Lemp MA, et al. 2015. "Clinical guidelines for management of dry eye associated with Sjögren's disease." *Ocul Surf* 13(2):118-32. doi: 10.1016/j.jtos.2014.12.001. PubMed PMID: 25881996.

- Fox PC, Atkinson JC, Macynski AA, et al. 1991. "Pilocarpine treatment of salivary gland hypofunction and dry mouth (xerostomia)." *Arch Intern Med* 151:1149-1152.

- Fox PC, Busch KA, Baum BJ. 1987. "Subjective reports of xerostomia and objective measures of salivary gland performance." *J Am Dent Assoc* 115:581–4.

- Fox PC. 2007. "Autoimmune diseases and Sjögren's syndrome: an autoimmune exocrinopathy." *Ann N Y Acad Sci* 1098:15-21.

- Gordan VV, Blaser PK, Watson RE, Mjor IA, McEdward DL, Sensi LG, et al. 2014. "A clinical evaluation of a giomer restorative system containing surface prereacted glass ionomer filler: results from a 13-year recall examination." *J Am Dent Assoc* 145(10):1036-43. doi: 10.14219/jada.2014.57. PubMed PMID: 25270702.

- Graziano TS, Calil CM, Sartoratto A, Franco GC, Groppo FC, Cogo-Muller K. 2016. "In vitro effects of Melaleuca alternifolia essential oil on growth and production of volatile sulphur compounds by oral bacteria." *J Appl Oral Sci* 24(6):582-9. doi: 10.1590/1678-775720160044. PubMed PMID: 28076463; PubMed Central PMCID: PMCPMC5404886.

- Grushka M, Ching V, Epstein J. 2006. "Burning mouth syndrome." *Adv Otorhinolaryngol* 63:278-87.

- Guggenheimer J, Moore PA. 2003. "Xerostomia: Etiology, recognition and treatment." *J Am Dent Assoc* 134:61-69.

- Haag DG, Peres KG, Balasubramanian M, Brennan DS. 2017. "Oral Conditions and Health-Related Quality of Life: A Systematic Review." *J Dent Res* 96:864-874.

- Hanada M, Koda H, Onaga K, Tanaka K, Okabayashi T, Itoh T, et al. 2003. "Portable oral malodor analyzer using highly sensitive In2O3 gas sensor combined with a simple gas chromatography system." *Anal Chim Acta* 475(1-2):27-35. Epub 29 Oct 2002. doi: 10.1016/S0003-2670(02)01038-3.

- Hannig M, Hannig C. 2014. "The pellicle and erosion." *Monogr Oral Sci* 25:206-14.

- Hara AT, Zero DT, 2014. "The Potential of Saliva in Protecting against Dental Erosion." *Monogr Oral Sci* 25:197-205.

- Haraszthy VI, Zambon JJ, Sreenivasan PK, et al. 2007. "Identification of oral bacterial species associated with halitosis." *J Am Dent Assoc* 138:1113-20.

- Haveman CW, Summitt JB, Burgess JO, Carlson K. 2003. "Three restorative materials and topical fluoride gel used in xerostomic patients: a clinical comparison." *J Am Dent Assoc* 134:177-84.

- Helmick CG, Felson DT, Lawrence RC, Gabriel S, Hirsch R, Kwoh CK, et al. 2008. "Estimates of the prevalence of arthritis and other rheumatic conditions in the United States. Part I." *Arthritis Rheum* 58(1):15-25. doi: 10.1002/art.23177. PubMed PMID: 18163481.

- Holbrook EH, Leopold DA. 2006. "An updated review of clinical olfaction." *Curr Opin Otolaryngol Head Neck Surg* 14:23-8.

- Horst JA, Ellenikiotis H, Milgrom PL. 2016. "UCSF Protocol for Caries Arrest Using Silver Diamine Fluoride: Rationale, Indications and Consent." *J Calif Dent Assoc* 44:16-28.

- Janket SJ, Jones JA, Rich S, Meurman J, Garcia R, Miller D. 2003. "Xerostomia medications and oral health: The Veterans Dental Study (Part I)." *Gerodontology* 20:41-49.

- Järvinen VK1, Rytömaa II, Heinonen OP. 1991. "Risk factors in dental erosion." *J Dent Res* 70:942-7.

- Jenson L, Budenz AW, Featherstone JBD, Ramos-Gomez F, Spolsky VW, Young DA. 2007. "Clinical Protocols for Caries Management by Risk Assessment." *J Calif Dent Assoc* 35:714-723.

- Joyston-Bechal S, Hayes K, Davenport ES, Hardie JM. 1992. Caries incidence, mutans streptococci and lactobacilli in irradiated patients during a 12-month preventive programme using chlorhexidine and fluoride. *Caries Res* 26:384-390.

- Korfage A, Raghoebar GM, Arends S, Meiners PM, Visser A, Kroese FG, et al. 2016. "Dental Implants in Patients with Sjögren's Syndrome." *Clin Implant Dent Relat Res* 18(5):937-45. doi: 10.1111/cid.12376. PubMed PMID: 26399938.Lal D, Hotaling AJ. Drooling. Curr Opin Otolaryngol Head Neck Surg 2006;14:381-6.

- LeBel G, Haas B, Adam AA, Veilleux MP, Lagha AB, Grenier D. 2017. "Effect of cinnamon (Cinnamomum verum) bark essential oil on the halitosis-associated bacterium Solobacterium moorei and in vitro cytotoxicity." *Arch Oral Biol* 83:97-104. doi: 10.1016/j.archoralbio.2017.07.005. PubMed PMID: 28743086.

- Leung WK, Dassanayake RS, Yau JY, Jin LJ, Yam WC, Samaranayake LP. 2000. "Oral colonization, phenotypic, and genotypic profiles of Candida species in irradiated, dentate, xerostomic nasopharyngeal carcinoma survivors." *J Clin Microbiol* 38:2219-26.

- Lim M, Mace A, Nouraei SA, Sandhu G. 2006. "Botulinum toxin in the management of sialorrhoea: a systematic review." *Clin Otolaryngol* 31:267-72.

- Lussi A, Carvalho TS. 2014. "Erosive Tooth Wear: A Multifactorial Condition of Growing Concern and Increasing Knowledge." *Monogr Oral Sci* 25:1-15.

- Malaty J, Malaty IA. 2013. "Smell and taste disorders in primary care." *Am Fam Physician* 88(12):852-9. PubMed PMID: 24364550.

- McCabe JF, Yan Z, Al Naimi OT, Mahmoud G, Rolland SL. 2011. "Smart materials in dentistry." *Aust Dent J* 56 Suppl 1:3-10. doi: 10.1111/j.1834-7819.2010.01291.x. PubMed PMID: 21564111.

- Meningaud JP, Pitak-Arnnop P, Chikhani L, Bertrand JC. 2006. "Drooling of saliva: a review of the etiology and management options." *Oral Surg Oral Med Oral Pathol Oral Radiol Endod* 101:48-57.

- Mott AE, Leopold DA. 1991. "Disorders in taste and smell." *Med Clin North Am* 75(6):1321-53. PubMed PMID: 1943323.

- Mouradian WE, Wehr E, Crall JJ. 2000. "Disparities in children's oral health and access to dental care." *J Am Med Assoc* 284:2625-2631.

- Nakhleh MK, Quatredeniers M, Haick H. 2017. "Detection of halitosis in breath: Between the past, present, and future." *Oral Dis* doi: 10.1111/odi.12699. PubMed PMID: 28622437.

- National Center for Health Statistics. 2015. "Health, United States, 2014: With Special Feature on Adults Aged 55–64." Hyattsville, MD.

- National Institute on Alcohol Abuse and Alcoholism. Drinking Levels Defined. https://www.niaaa.nih.gov/alcohol-health/overview-alcohol-consumption/moderate-binge-drinking

- Navazesh M, Christensen C, Brightman V. 1992. "Clinical criteria for the diagnosis of salivary gland hypofunction." *J Dent Res* 71:1363-1369.

- Navazesh M, Kumar SK. 2008. "Measuring salivary flow: challenges and opportunities." *J Am Dent Assoc* 139 Suppl:35S-40S. doi: 139/suppl_2/35S [pii].

- Nederfors T, Isaksson R, Mornstad H, Dahlof C. 1997. "Prevalence of perceived symptoms of dry mouth in an adult Swedish population-relation to age, sex and pharmacotherapy." *Community Dent Oral Epidemiol* 25:211-216.

- Nishihira J, Nishimura M, Tanaka A, Yamaguchi A, Taira T. 2017. "Effects of 4-week continuous ingestion of champignon extract on halitosis and body and fecal odor." *J Tradit Complement Med* 7(1):110-6. doi: 10.1016/j.jtcme.2015.11.002. PubMed PMID: 28053896; PubMed Central PMCID: PMCPMC5198824.

- Patil S, Acharya S, Hathiwala S, Singhal DK, Srinivasan SR, Khatri S. 2017. "Evaluation of the Efficacy of G32 (Commercially Available Ayurvedic Preparation) in Reducing Halitosis – A Randomized Controlled Trial." *J Clin Diagn Res* 11(9):ZC79-ZC83. doi: 10.7860/JCDR/2017/27380.10678. PubMed PMID: 29207840; PubMed Central PMCID: PMCPMC5713862.

- Porciani PF, Grandini S. 2016. "Effect of Green Tea-Added Tablets on Volatile Sulfur-Containing Compounds in the Oral Cavity." *J Clin Dent* 27(4):110-3. PubMed PMID: 28391664.

- Porter SR, Scully C. 2006. "Oral malodour (halitosis)." *BMJ* 333(7569):632-5. doi: 10.1136/bmj.38954.631968.AE. PubMed PMID: 16990322; PubMed Central PMCID: PMCPMC1570844.

- Rao AS, Kumar V. 2013. "Halitosis: A mirror of systemic and oral health." *IOSR Journal of Dental and Medical Sciences* 4(3):7-12.

- Rawal S, Hoffman HJ, Bainbridge KE, Huedo-Medina TB, Duffy VB. 2016. "Prevalence and Risk Factors of Self-Reported Smell and Taste Alterations: Results from the 2011-2012 US National Health and Nutrition Examination Survey (NHANES)." *Chem Senses* 41(1):69-76. doi: 10.1093/chemse/bjv057. PubMed PMID: 26487703; PubMed Central PMCID: PMCPMC4715252.

- Rosenberg M, Kulkarni GV, Bosy A, McCulloch CA. 1991. "Reproducibility and sensitivity of oral malodor measurements with a portable sulphide monitor." *J Dent Res* 70(11):1436-40. doi: 10.1177/00220345910700110801. PubMed PMID: 1960254.

- Sanz M, Roldan S, Herrera D. 2001. "Fundamentals of breath malodour." *J Contemp Dent Pract* 2(4):1-17. PubMed PMID: 12167916.

- Scully C. 2003. "Drug effects on salivary glands: dry mouth." *Oral Dis* 9(4):165-76. PubMed PMID: 12974516.

- Scully C, Greenman J. 2012. "Halitology (breath odour: aetiopathogenesis and management)." *Oral Dis* 18(4):333-45. doi: 10.1111/j.1601-0825.2011.01890.x. PubMed PMID: 22277019.

- Seiberling KA, Conley DB. 2004. "Aging and olfactory and taste function." *Otolaryngol Clin N Am* 37:1209-1228.

- Shellis RP, Addy M. 2014. "The interactions between attrition, abrasion and erosion in tooth wear." *Monogr Oral Sci* 25:32-45.

- Shiboski CH, Shiboski SC, Seror R, Criswell LA, Labetoulle M, Lietman TM, et al. 2017. "American College of Rheumatology/European League Against Rheumatism classification criteria for primary Sjögren's syndrome: A consensus and data-driven methodology involving three international patient cohorts." *Ann Rheum Dis* 76(1):9-16. doi: 10.1136/annrheumdis-2016-210571. PubMed PMID: 27789466.

- Shimura M, Yasuno Y, Iwakura M, Shimada Y, Sakai S, Suzuki K, et al. 1996. "A new monitor with a zinc-oxide thin film semiconductor sensor for the measurement of volatile sulfur compounds in mouth air." *J Periodontol* 67(4):396-402. doi: 10.1902/jop.1996.67.4.396. PubMed PMID: 8708966.

- Silva MF, Leite FRM, Ferreira LB, Pola NM, Scannapieco FA, Demarco FF, et al. 2018. "Estimated prevalence of halitosis: a systematic review and meta-regression analysis." *Clin Oral Investig* 22(1):47-55. doi: 10.1007/s00784-017-2164-5. PubMed PMID: 28676903.

- Sterer N, Rosenberg M. 2011. *Breath Odors of Nasal and Pharyngeal Origin. Breath Odors: Origin, Diagnosis, and Management.* p. 41-6. Springer-Verlag Berlin Heidelberg.

- Suh KI, Lee JY, Chung JW, Kim YK, Kho HS. 2007. "Relationship between salivary flow rate and clinical symptoms and behaviours in patients with dry mouth." *J Oral Rehabil* 34:739-44.

- Thanou-Stavraki A, James JA. 2008. "Primary Sjögren's syndrome: current and prospective therapies." *Semin Arthritis Rheum* 37:273-92.

- van Bijsterveld OP. 1969. "Diagnostic tests in the Sicca Syndrome." *Arch Ophthalmol* 82(1):10-4.

- van den Broek AM, Feenstra L, de Baat C. 2008. A review of the current literature on management of halitosis. *Oral Dis* 14:30-9.

- Villa A, Wolff A, Aframian D, Vissink A, Ekström J, Proctor G, McGowan R, Narayana N, Aliko A, Sia YW, Joshi RK, Jensen SB, Kerr AR, Dawes C, Pedersen AM. 2015. "World Workshop on Oral Medicine VI: a systematic review of medication-induced salivary gland dysfunction: prevalence, diagnosis, and treatment." *Clin Oral Investig* 19:1563-80.

- Vivino FB, Carsons SE, Foulks G, Daniels TE, Parke A, Brennan MT, et al. 2016. "New Treatment Guidelines for Sjögren's Disease." *Rheum Dis Clin North Am* 42(3):531-51. doi: 10.1016/j.rdc.2016.03.010. PubMed PMID: 27431353.

- Whitcher JP, Shiboski CH, Shiboski SC, Heidenreich AM, Kitagawa K, Zhang S, et al. 2010. "A simplified quantitative method for assessing keratoconjunctivitis sicca from the Sjögren's Syndrome International Registry." *Am J Ophthalmol* 149(3):405-15. doi: 10.1016/j.ajo.2009.09.013. PubMed PMID: 20035924; PubMed Central PMCID: PMCPMC3459675.

- Yoo JI, Shin IS, Jeon JG, Yang YM, Kim JG, Lee DW. 2017. "The Effect of Probiotics on Halitosis: a Systematic Review and Meta-analysis." *Probiotics Antimicrob Proteins* doi: 10.1007/s12602-017-9351-1. PubMed PMID: 29168154.

- Young DA, Novy BB, Zeller GG, Hale R, Hart TC, Truelove EL. 2015. "The American Dental Association Caries Classification System for clinical practice: a report of the American Dental Association Council on Scientific Affairs." *J Am Dent Assoc* 146:79-86.

- Zero DT, Brennan MT, Daniels TE, Papas A, Stewart C, Pinto A, et al. 2016. "Clinical practice guidelines for oral management of Sjögren's disease: Dental caries prevention." *J Am Dent Assoc* 147(4):295-305. doi: 10.1016/j.adaj.2015.11.008. PubMed PMID: 26762707.

- Zou YM, Lu D, Liu LP, Zhang HH, Zhou YY. 2016. Olfactory dysfunction in Alzheimer's disease. *Neuropsychiatr Dis Treat.* 12:869-75. doi: 10.2147/NDT.S104886. PubMed PMID: 27143888; PubMed Central PMCID: PMCPMC4841431.

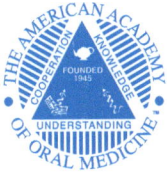

The American Academy of Oral Medicine
2150 N. 107th St., Suite 205
Seattle, Washington 98133
PHONE: (206) 209-5279 · EMAIL: info@aaom.com

Application for AAOM Membership

ELIGIBILITY FOR MEMBERSHIP

1. Nominee for **Regular Membership** shall be a graduate of an accredited Dental School or Medicine School and shall be a member of his/her representative National Society and shall pursue special interest or accomplishment in the field of Oral Medicine.

2. Nominee for **Affiliate Membership** (student) shall be a graduate of an accredited Dental or Medical School and shall be a member of his/her representative National Society and currently in training in a Postdoctoral program.

3. Nominee for **Student Membership** shall be a student currently enrolled in a pre-doctoral program in an accredited dental or medical school. Students are those seeking a DDS, DMD or MD degree.

4. The fiscal year for dues starts January 1.

5. After acceptance into the Academy, Active Membership dues are paid annually and include a subscription to ORAL SURGERY, ORAL MEDICINE, ORAL PATHOLOGY, ORAL RADIOLOGY, and ENDODONTOLOGY.

6. Please see the AAOM website for more membership information and how to apply: www.aaom.com.